Caring
for your
Child

a complete
medical
guide

BY
WILLIAM E. HOMAN, M.D.
& THE EDITORS OF CONSUMER GUIDE®

HARMONY BOOKS/NEW YORK

CONTENTS

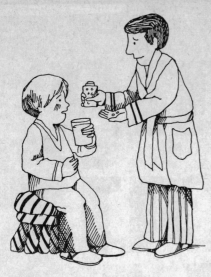

Louis Weber, President
Publications International Ltd.
3841 West Oakton Street
Skokie, Illinois 60076

Permission is never granted for commercial purposes.

Published by
Harmony Books,
a division of Crown Publishers, Inc.
One Park Avenue
New York, New York 10016

Manufactured in the United States of America
1 2 3 4 5 6 7 8 9 10

Library of Congress Cataloging in Publication Data:

Homan, William E.   1919-
    Caring for your child.

    Includes index.
    1. Children—Diseases—Dictionaries. 2.
Children—Wounds and injuries—Dictionaries. I.
Consumer guide. II. Title.
RJ61.H785   618.9'2   79-8044
ISBN 0-517-53957-8
ISBN 0-517-53910-1 pbk.

Consulting Editor: Karen M. Sandrick

Illustrations: Nan Brooks

CONTENTS

CONTENTS

NOTICE

Childhood illnesses can be perplexing to a distraught parent. The infant's first sniffle, an unexplained rash, the newborn's colicky distress, all can make a parent anxious not only to relieve the child's discomfort but also to make sure that the ailment is not a signal of serious illness. Does the child's fever indicate a sore throat, infectious mononucleosis, or a myriad of other diseases in which fever is present?

A minor cut can easily be diagnosed by the parent, and it can be dealt with appropriately without hesitation. But, if the child has a serious fall and injures his arm, how can the parent tell if it's a fracture? If the child is hit on the head with a ball, could he have a concussion? If a burn is more than minor, can the parent treat it, or should the child be taken to a health care facility?

Such questions can cause the anxious parent serious concern, sometimes even panic. CARING FOR YOUR CHILD urges parents to plan ahead for ailments that can and do occur at any time. Some problems can be treated at home; others demand a doctor's care. The informed parent has a far better chance of promptly identifying which is which than does one who is unprepared. It is difficult to second guess what a child may get into that will cause an injury, which viruses he may be exposed to, when he will come down with a bad sore throat. The parent who can consult CARING FOR YOUR CHILD will know what symptoms to look for to judge the severity of a cough, what he can do at home to comfort the child, when he must consult a doctor.

William Homan, MD, a pediatrician with years of experience, with the help of the editors of CONSUMER GUIDE®, has gathered together information on over 150 common problems that afflict children from infancy through adolescence. You may have already had to deal with some of these; without a doubt you will have to deal with others in the future.

Each profile covers a single disease or condition and includes a description that will aid the parent in identifying the probable cause of the problem. The parent will find the descriptions helpful in distinguishing impetigo from ringworm, colic from teething pains. Each description is written to reassure the parent if the condition tends to be self-correcting, to alert the parent if serious complications are possible.

How is the diagnosis for a single disease confirmed? You'll find out it you can diagnose the problem at home, if it must be done in the doctor's office, or if laboratory tests or

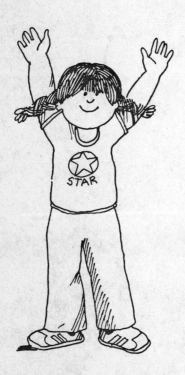
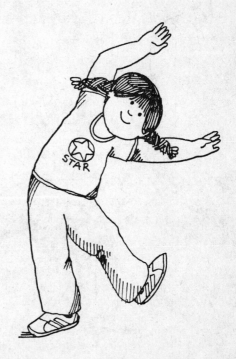

INTRODUCTION

screenings are necessary.

If home treatment is possible or helpful, CARING FOR YOUR CHILD tells you what you can do: how to make your child more comfortable when he has a cold, the emergency measures necessary if he has swallowed poison or is choking on a bone. The Home Treatment section of each entry also describes the home therapy your doctor may prescribe—a course of drugs or a special diet.

Precautions that should be taken to protect your child are also included. The precautions will not only help to prevent your child from getting ill, but will also alert you to possible complications, drug misuse, and those situations in which you must see the doctor.

The Doctor's Treatment section of each entry is not a recommended treatment but rather an overall view of what your doctor might find necessary—including laboratory tests, X rays, drug therapy, hospitalization for intravenous feedings, and surgery. Reading this section will prepare you by letting you know what to expect from your office visit.

By reading these entries, you can become familiar with what you can do to avoid serious illness and when you must seek medical aid. As a home medical text, CARING FOR YOUR CHILD will also guide you in those steps that should *not* be taken.

CARING FOR YOUR CHILD will guide you in making decisions about medical care—it explains how to choose the best doctor for your child, whether a pediatrician or a family physician, and how to develop a good working partnership. A chapter tells which immunizations are necessary, at what age they should be administered, and whether boosters are necessary to provide your child lifelong protection.

What should you keep in your home medicine chest to be ready to deal with most any situation? CARING FOR YOUR CHILD tells you what to include, and how to use the medications. Of course you should consult your own doctor for recommendations on medications and dosages.

Many parents have trouble administering drugs. CARING FOR YOUR CHILD tells you how to give the proper amount of medication to a child, what "four times a day" means, and why it's important that you continue treatment for as long as the doctor prescribes, even if your child's symptoms do clear up earlier.

Sometimes it is necessary to use extraordinary measures to get an uncooperative child to take his medicine. CARING FOR YOUR CHILD tells how to use a dropper for liquid

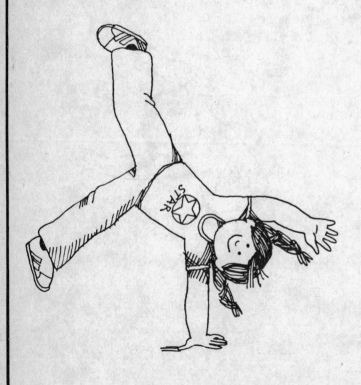
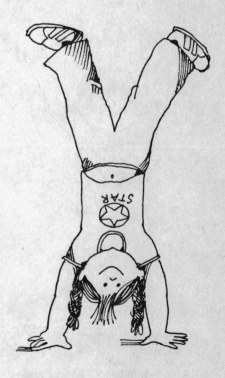

INTRODUCTION

medicine for a very young child and a sweet disguise for the unpalatable potion, how to mash a bulky tablet, how to teach a child to swallow a pill, when to use rectal medications, and even how to "mummy" a terrified child when no other method seems to work.

The most common symptoms of childhood illness are explained in chapters on fever and lymph nodes. Parents who panic when their child has a fever will find that, in many cases, their fears are unfounded. Fever is not a reliable indicator of the severity of the illness, but a signal that the child is sick. It is recommended that you reduce the fever to make the child comfortable, but not fight the fever in the mistaken belief that you are treating the illness.

Lymph nodes become swollen and tender when they become infected. Swollen "glands," therefore, do indicate that your child is fighting an infection. CARING FOR YOUR CHILD offers a detailed description of what these infection-fighting nodes are, how they work, and how they can be used to help diagnose illness.

CARING FOR YOUR CHILD includes a "Chart of Symptoms" to help you discern the possible causes of your child's malady. It lists the principal symptoms of common childhood diseases in a handy chart form. Use the chart

when you are unsure what disease your child may have.

CARING FOR YOUR CHILD is written in easy to understand language and it will relieve you of much of the anxiety that comes with having a sick child. You'll find it a reliable aid in helping to decide whether to call the doctor, go to the emergency room, or treat the child at home. Of course, you must consult your doctor about drug usage or any unusual symptoms your child has.

The editors of CONSUMER GUIDE® suggest that you take an hour or so to browse through this book before a specific need arises. You want to know beforehand how to deal with an emergency situation such as choking or poisoning. And you want to be alert to those early warning symptoms that may indicate serious illness. By taking the time to become familiar with this book, you will be able to use the information contained herein wisely and well when it's needed.

Children do get sick. They fall and cut themselves; they pick up germs; they suffer from allergies, and headaches, and pains in the joints. And every parent wants to be able to help his children feel better faster and to guard them from serious illness. CARING FOR YOUR CHILD can be a real tool for every parent.

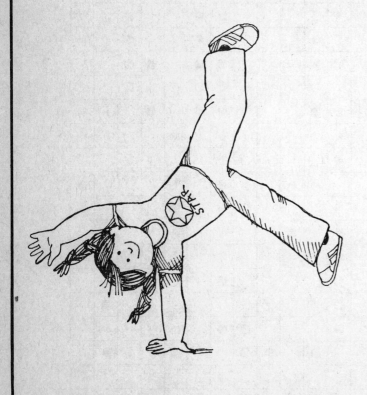
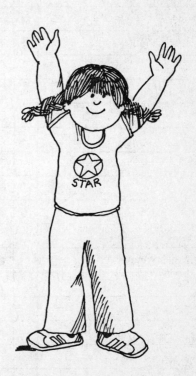

CHART OF SYMPTOMS

Here are some common childhood diseases (vertical column) and their symptoms (across the top). **Key** symptoms are indicated by a solid dot; **possible** symptoms are indicated by an open dot. To use this chart run your finger down the columns that correspond to each of your child's symptoms, and read the diseases (to the left) which cause each symptom. By a process of elimination you should be able to zero in on the possible causes of your child's illness. Then, turn to the section of the book relating to the various diseases. There you'll find both the information you need to further narrow down the diagnosis and the treatment recommended to relieve distress.

Signs and Symptoms

Diseases	Unconsciousness	Vomiting	Visible Deformity	Tenderness	Rash	Pain	Noisy Breathing	Loss of Function	Itching	Headache	Fever	Difficulty Breathing	Diarrhea	Cough	Blueness	Abnormal Discharge	Abnormal Behavior
Appendicitis		○		●		●					●		○				
Arthritis			○	○	○	●		●			○						
Asthma		○					●					●		●	○		
Blood Poisoning		○		●						○	●						
Boils				●		●					○						
Botulism		●				●						●	●				
Bronchiolitis							●				●	○		●	○		
Bronchitis							○	○			●	○		●			
Chicken Pox					●				●	○	●						
Common Cold							○	○		○	●			●	○		
Concussion	●	●						○		●	○						●
Convulsions with Fever	●						○			●	●			●			
Convulsions without Fever	●					●			○		●			●			
Croup		○			○	●				●	●			●	○		
Cystic Fibrosis							○				●	○	○	●	○		
Diphtheria						●	●			●	●			●			
Dysentery		○		○		●					●		●				
Earaches		○		●		●				○	○						
Encephalitis	○	●								●	●						●
Food Poisoning		●				●				○	●		●				
Fractures			●	●		●		●									
Gastroenteritis, Acute		●		○		●					●		●				
Glands, Swollen			●	○		○					●						
Gonorrhea						○										●	
Hand, Foot, & Mouth Disease				○	●	●				○	●						
Hay Fever							○		●	○						●	
Hepatitis		○				○			○	○	●						
Hernia			●	○		○											

● Key Symptoms   ○ Possible Symptoms

CHART OF SYMPTOMS

Diseases	Unconsciousness	Vomiting	Visible Deformity	Tenderness	Rash	Pain	Noisy Breathing	Loss of Function	Itching	Headache	Fever	Difficulty Breathing	Diarrhea	Cough	Blueness	Abnormal Discharge	Abnormal Behavior
Herpes Simplex					○	●					○						
Hypertension										○							
Impetigo				●					○								
Infectious Mononucleosis					○	●				○	●						
Influenza		○				●				○	●		○	●			
Intestinal Allergies		○		○		●			○				●				
Laryngitis					○	○				○				●			
Leukemia					○	○					●						
Measles		○			●				○	○	●			●			
Meningitis	○	●			○					●	●						●
Mumps		○	●	●		●				○	●						
Nephritis	○	○								○	●						
Pinworms						○			●								
Pneumonia		○				○	○			○	●	●		●	○		
Poisoning	○	○				○	○			○		○	○	○	○		○
Polio		○				●		●		○	●	○					
Rocky Mountain Spotted Fever	○				●	●				○	●						
Roseola	○				●						●						
Rubella					●						●						
Scabies					●				●								
Sinusitis				●		●				●	●			●		○	
Sore Throat		○		○	○	●	○			○	●			○			
Stomach Ache, Acute		○		○		●					○		○				
Stomach Ache, Chronic		○		○		●					○		○				
Strep Throat		○		○	○	●	○			○	●			○		○	
Swimmer's Ear				●		●		○	○		○						●
Tetanus	●					●		○		○	●	●				○	
Tonsillitis		○		○	○	●	○			○	●			○			
Ulcers		○		○		●											
Urinary Tract Infections		○		○		○					●						
Viruses		○			○	○	○			○	●	○	○	○			
Whooping Cough		●									●			●	○		

● *Key Symptoms* ○ *Possible Symptoms*

THE PARENT/PHYSICIAN PARTNERSHIP

Raising a child properly to good emotional and physical health is a tough job that requires cooperation and love from all the child's guardians. A trained and experienced person, who is a reliable and sympathetic source of information and suggestions, can help immeasurably. Your child's doctor should be that person. But he or she should not take the child's rearing out of your hands by making all decisions for you or by dictating a single course of action without adequate explanation. Only you, the parent, can make judgments concerning what is best for your child—judgments based on knowing the important facts and alternatives. Above all else, you should feel comfortable talking to your child's doctor and following his or her advice.

Whom to Choose. To get the best from your child's doctor, you must first select the best

doctor for your child. A pediatrician sees only children and has had three to five years post-doctoral training in the special emotional, physical, and educational needs of young people. A family physician usually has had nearly as much training, but it has not been devoted exclusively to children. The best pediatrician in the country should know more about children than the best family doctor, but neither will know everything about all children. A family doctor who is interested in children—in your child in particular—and with whom you feel safe and comfortable may be a better choice for you than a pediatrician with whom you can't relate.

There are several ways to go about finding a physician for your family. If you are an expectant mother, your obstetrician can recommend a number of local pediatricians and

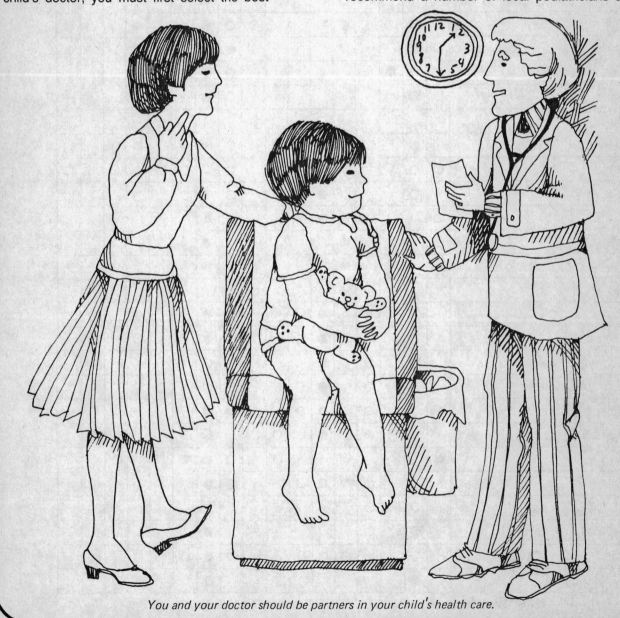

You and your doctor should be partners in your child's health care.

THE PARENT/PHYSICIAN PARTNERSHIP

family physicians from which to choose. If you are new to an area you may consult a neighbor who has children or call the local hospital or branch of the state medical society. An initial phone call and visit to a doctor should determine whether or not that physician is right for you and your child. Once you find a doctor with whom you feel confident, there are a number of ways you can help promote your child's good care.

Take Time to Make Time. A common cause of communication breakdown between parent and physician is the complaint: "My doctor didn't give me enough time to ask all my questions!" This conflict can be avoided if, when you make an appointment, you let the receptionist know what the visit is for and that you will need extra time to discuss this (or another) problem with the doctor. If possible, you should mention your problems in advance so the doctor can consider them before seeing your child. The following classic requests, sprung on the doctor during a 15-minute appointment for a sore throat or a case of the chicken pox, may take attention away from the initial reason for the visit: "As long as I'm here, I'd like to ask you about: John's poor performance in school this year and last; Sarah's rash; Sue's stomach ache, which she's had every night for the past six months; Tom's bedwetting..." and so on. A hurried doctor might be tempted to offer you brief, off-the-cuff advice to ease your mind and to keep up with his schedule, but this approach leaves you cheated and the doctor feeling guilty. Allow your doctor time to treat one thing at a time.

With rare exception, children's doctors are glad to allow time to discuss complicated problems . . . if they are forewarned. If you feel rushed during your appointment, simply request time to discuss the situation or ask to come back when more time is available.

Be Specific. When you call, don't leave it up to your doctor to guess whether you want telephone advice or an office visit. If the doctor feels that a trip to the office is unnecessary—a waste of your money and the doctor's time—you'll be told why. But the decision is yours. It's your child and your money, and most doctors don't want to decide for you. Also, when you call, be sure to notify your doctor of any medications your child is allergic to or whether there are other special circumstances to be considered.

Ask Questions. If a doctor's advice seems wrong to you or is hard to follow, ask "Why?" and "What are the alternatives?" If you don't like the answers, try another doctor, but don't argue. You may get what you want, but it may be second- or third-best for your child.

House Calls. Whether or not your doctor makes house calls should not be a criterion by which to judge professional ability. All capable doctors are available promptly in an emergency. But good doctors have learned that it is a sham to examine a sick child in a poorly lighted bedroom without adequate equipment available. More wrong diagnoses have been made in this way than in any other. It's far better to take a sick child to an office with the proper facilities where a correct diagnosis is a hundredfold more likely, than to request a house call.

Before You Call. Be prepared to answer questions when you phone your doctor for advice. You will get much better service if you have the following at the tip of your tongue:

- your child's approximate weight (medications are given by weight);
- your child's temperature (take it by thermometer; don't guess);
- what medicines the child is allergic to;
- what illnesses the child has been exposed to recently; and
- the druggist's name and telephone number and the hours the pharmacy is open (days, nights, weekends, and holidays).

Finally, have paper and pencil at hand to write down any instructions the doctor might give you.

Health Forms. Before submitting camp and school forms and health insurance claims, fill in whatever is required on your part and as much other information as you can. Grant your doctor time to practice his profession not his penmanship.

A Second Opinion. If you want another doctor's opinion, ask for a consultation. No physician relishes assuming all the responsibility for a difficult case. Allow the doctor you trust to suggest the names of possible consultants. You can trust the competence of the consultant as you do your own doctor's.

Satisfaction Guaranteed. Let your doctor know when you are displeased with the service you are receiving. If it can be changed to better suit your needs, it will be. If not, find another physician.

As there are good and bad lawyers, engineers, teachers, and parents, there are also good and bad doctors. But a physician's failure to please you may be due to many factors other than professional inadequacy. To ensure a good relationship and the best possible care for your child, select your doctor carefully and communicate openly. Your child's good health care depends on your physician and you.

FEVER

There is a popular fallacy which sets forth that the higher the fever, the sicker the child. It is also believed that fever is a child's enemy, that it should be fought and the temperature brought to normal.

The fact is that children past early infancy tend to develop high fevers with little provocation. Relatively harmless illnesses like roseola often cause temperatures as high as 106°F, whereas many lethal diseases, such as leukemia and polio, may cause slight or no temperature deviations at all.

A child is as seriously sick as the illness warrants, not as a thermometer registers. A child with pneumonia or meningitis and a fever of 104°F is still as ill after the temperature is artificially reduced to normal. A child with a strep throat and 101°F fever is no less threatened than the same child with a strep throat and a temperature of 104°F. Prostration, disorientation, difficulty in breathing, and other symptoms are means to decide the illness's severity, not the degree of fever.

Fever: Friend and Foe. You should first regard a fever as a child's friend rather than an enemy. A fever is an early warning signal that a child is ill and that you must look to find a cause. It is also a helpful barometer to judge, together with other symptoms, when an illness is ending. The course of a fever indicates whether or not an antibiotic is working effectively. It speeds up the body's metabolic processes (possibly including its immunizing mechanisms) and in some instances may help the body's defenses overcome an illness. Finally, the pattern of daily fluctuations in a fever may be characteristic of particular illnesses and aid the parent or physician in making a correct diagnosis.

A high fever does have disadvantages, however. It makes a child feel bad and, as it develops, causes chills. If a fever continues for days, it will debilitate a child and cause weakness and the need for a longer recuperation period. In susceptible younger children a fever may precipitate convulsions (see Convulsions with Fever). For all these reasons, it is sensible to reduce a fever. But it is important not to confuse treating the fever with treating the illness and not to panic as a fever rises or to harm the child in your anxiety to fight the fever.

A Matter of Degree. At any given moment, different parts of the body are at different temperatures. Moreover, normal temperatures vary as much as two to three degrees Fahrenheit over the course of a day even when a child is healthy. A rectal temperature of 99.8°F or less, an oral temperature of 98.6°F or below, and an armpit temperature, though the least accurate, of 98°F or less are all considered normal.

Despite these variances, all thermometers are marked to indicate 98.6°F as normal. A rectal thermometer differs from an oral one only in having a more rugged bulb. (The most practical instrument for home use is a stubby bulb thermometer, which can be used to take a child's temperature in either of the preferred ways.)

Any type of thermometer—rectal, stubby, or oral—can be used to take a rectal temperature. If the oral one is pressed into service, extra care must be taken because of its more pointed and fragile bulb. For the most reliable readings at any age, the rectal thermometer is recommended, although it takes a bit more time for a fever to register.

Taking the Temperature. No one can estimate the degree of a fever by touch; not even a mother. If your child feels warm or appears ill, you must use a thermometer to attain the information you and your doctor need to treat the child.

Read the thermometer before inserting it to be certain the mercury column is below 98.6°F and the bulb is intact. Spread the child's buttocks widely enough with the thumb and forefinger of one hand so the anal opening is clearly visible. Lubricate the bulb and insert it gently into the center of the anus. There should be no pain or discomfort. (Only the bulb portion of the thermometer needs to be inserted for the two to three minutes required to obtain an accurate reading.)

You can sufficiently restrain a baby by placing him or her face down on a solid surface and putting the heel of your hand firmly on the lower back. An uncooperative toddler can be firmly clasped between your thighs and bent forward over one leg in a position to expose the target.

Although less reliable, an oral reading will suffice and can be taken in a child who is old enough to hold the bulb of the thermometer under the tongue for three minutes. (If a child accidentally swallows the mercury in the thermometer, don't fret. Thermometers contain elemental mercury, a nonpoisonous and harmless form of the metal.)

Care of Your Thermometer. After each use, the thermometer should be shaken down below "normal" and washed with soap and cold water. To sterilize it, you may soak the thermometer in an alcohol solution before storing it in its case. Place it back in the medicine cabinet where it will be handy the next time you need it.

"But my child won't let me take his

temperature," some parents report. Here's an opportunity to teach a child one of the important lessons he needs to get along in the world: self-control.

Self-control is merely the internalization of the knowledge that one's actions are capable of being controlled. You demonstrate this to your young child by restraining him from dashing into the path of a truck, taking a hatchet to a peer, or the TV set...and by firmly insisting that he allow you to take his temperature. A calm but determined approach to all of these situations can reassure the child that you are a capable parent upon whose wisdom, strength, and judgment he can depend for guidance and support.

Treatment of Fever. The most reliable medications for lowering fever are aspirin and acetaminophen, a pain reliever found in some over-the-counter preparations. Oral preparations are best, but rectal suppositories are permissible if a child is vomiting or unconscious (see Convulsions with Fever). Sixty milligrams of either may be given for every 12 pounds of the child's weight and repeated every four

hours if necessary. This formula works out to one children's aspirin for every 15 pounds of weight. If the fever does not respond to either aspirin or acetaminophen, the drugs may be given together in the same dose. Keep a feverish child lightly clothed or covered to allow the body heat to escape. This, too, will help lower a fever.

Other methods of reducing a fever include placing the child in a cool bath; encasing the nude child in a wet sheet; washing the child down from chin to toe with rubbing alcohol diluted with an equal amount of water; administering a cold enema; and packing ice bags around the child's body. These methods are seldom necessary, not recommended, and are generally resisted by the child. And none is obligatory unless the temperature goes over 106°F for a sustained period. If the temperature rises that high, the child is better off under the care of a doctor who can employ a thermostatically controlled cooling device to lower the temperature.

Fever is a tool. Learn to use it properly to make your child well again.

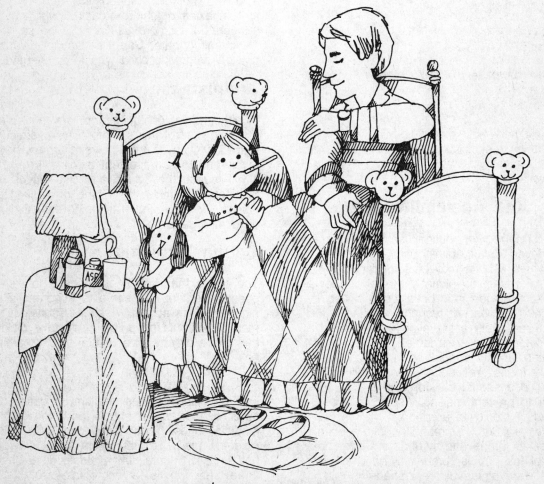

Lower a child's fever with aspirin or acetaminophen.

THE PEDIATRIC MEDICINE CHEST

The contents of a medicine chest may be as simple or as elaborate as the special needs of your child and the availability of professional medical services. Be sure to consult your doctor before purchasing and administering any medications. In average circumstances, the following list of 20 items should meet all your needs in semi-emergency situations until you can reach your pharmacy. All items should be clearly labelled in their original containers with child-proof tops and should be stored out of reach of even the most inquisitive young child. (Even if you have no children of your own, be careful to store things away from visiting friends' offspring.)

Recommended Contents:

acetaminophen
adhesive bandages (assorted sizes)
adhesive tape
antiemetic
antihistamine
antiseptic solution
aspirin
burn ointment
codeine
cough medicine
decongestant
emetic
knitted roller bandage
lubricant
nasal aspirator
nose drops
sterile gauze pads
steristrips
steroid
thermometer

Aspirin And Acetaminophen

Aspirin is preferred for routine use to relieve pain and fever. But acetaminophen should be available when a child may be intolerant of aspirin or when aspirin alone does not control a fever. Acetaminophen may be given with aspirin for a fever that does not respond to either medicine alone. Both are available as flavored, chewable tablets and adult tablets, as rectal suppositories, and in various strengths. Suppository forms are useful when a child is vomiting. These should be stored in a refrigerator to prevent melting. Aspirin may be crushed and mixed with a spoonful of applesauce, jelly, or ice cream. Acetaminophen also comes as drops and syrup. **Caution:** The strengths of the popular brands differ; check the label. Be aware of the different strengths and

administer only in recommended dosages.

Codeine

Severe earaches, toothaches, and other pains that are not affected by aspirin or acetaminophen alone will respond if codeine is added. A liquid preparation of acetaminophen and codeine is sold by prescription, but a simple way to keep a small supply of codeine on hand for emergencies is to buy a cough medicine that contains codeine. One teaspoonful has one-sixth grain (10 mg) of codeine. It should be used only as a temporary measure, until professional help can be obtained. Codeine should never be given for abdominal pain that might be appendicitis.

Antiemetic

An antiemetic is a drug that suppresses nausea, vomiting, and dizziness. Dimenhydrinate is one such drug to help your child get through a miserable night. It can also serve as a mild sedative. Dimenhydrinate is sold as a liquid and a tablet. The rectal suppository form of promethazine or chlorpromazine, which must be refrigerated, is more useful than the same form of dimenhydrinate. **Caution:** Do not give any antinauseant to a child who is disoriented.

Antihistamine

In either tablet or liquid form, any antihistamine will help control the symptoms of allergic reactions such as hives, eye allergies, hay fever, and to some extent asthma. In addition it will reduce the itching and swelling of insect bites and minimize the itching of chicken pox, poison ivy, and other rashes. It can also serve as a mild sedative.

Cough Medicine

The cough medicine kept on hand for its codeine content can serve to suppress a severe night cough. **Caution:** A suppressant cough medicine should never be given to a child who has croup or any type of hindered breathing.

Emetic

This medicine induces vomiting in cases of swallowed poison. It should be in every medicine chest. Syrup of ipecac is recommended. It's convenient to have two small bottles, each containing a single dose of two to three teaspoonfuls for immediate use.

THE PEDIATRIC MEDICINE CHEST

Nose Drops, Nasal Aspirator, And Decongestant

Along with aspirin, acetaminophen, and cough medicine, these items are useful in treating the symptoms of common colds.

Steroid

Steroids are dangerous if used regularly for a week or more and if used in the presence of high blood pressure, stomach ulcers, tuberculosis, chicken pox, and some other illnesses. However, a few doses of a steroid are safe and can offer immediate relief. They are helpful in cases of hives, hay fever, croup, reactions to insect bites, sun poisoning, poison ivy, and asthma. Steroids are best used for the condition for which they are prescribed; they are not to be misused. Discuss with your doctor the advisability of keeping a few doses of a liquid or tablet steroid on hand.

Thermometer And Lubricant

A multipurpose, stubby-bulb thermometer, which can be used orally or rectally, is most practical. Any lubricating ointment will serve to grease a thermometer for rectal use, but a water-soluble gel is superior because it readily washes off in cold water.

Additions

Antiseptic solution, burn ointment, sterile gauze pads (2x2 and 3x3 inches), rolls of knitted bandage (2-inch and 3-inch), adhesive tape (¼ inch), steristrips, and adhesive bandages of assorted sizes—all are useful in treating minor accidents properly.

Related Topics: Burns, Common Cold, Coughs, Cuts, Eye Allergies, Hay Fever, Hives, Insect Bites, Poisoning, Scrapes, Vomiting

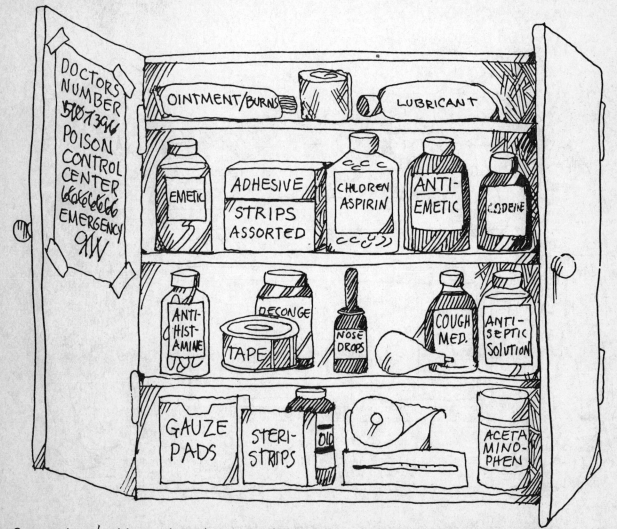

Get your doctor's advice on what to keep in your home medicine chest and on how to use the medications you keep.

IMMUNIZATIONS

All children should be properly immunized against seven potentially devastating diseases: diphtheria, tetanus, whooping cough (pertussis), polio, measles, mumps, and rubella. Surveys repeatedly indicate that almost 50 percent of American children are inadequately protected against these illnesses.

Two misconceptions cause this neglect. First, there is the belief that polio, diphtheria, and whooping cough are extinct illnesses; and second, there is ignorance of the dangers inherent in these diseases. Children die or are permanently disabled every year from these seven preventable diseases. Because the statistics indicate that there are children in danger of these illnesses, your child can become exposed. The following chapters detail the serious results of these diseases. The following pages indicate the ease with which they can be prevented.

Diphtheria, Tetanus, and Whooping Cough (Pertussis)

Infants require three injections of DTP (diphtheria, tetanus, pertussis) vaccine by age six months—starting at two months of age, and administered every other month. Following this initial series, they need a booster shot of DTP at age 18 to 24 months, and again at age four to six years. Thereafter, a booster shot of only diphtheria-tetanus vaccine is necessary every five to ten years for life.

Diphtheria. Cases of diphtheria are reported

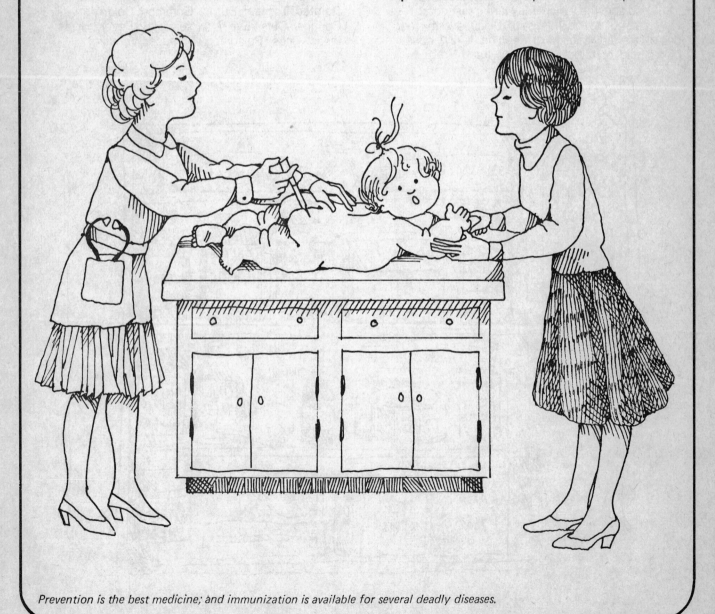

Prevention is the best medicine; and immunization is available for several deadly diseases.

in every state every year. For every case reported there are many persons who are carriers of diphtheria. Before the general use of diphtheria toxoid was introduced 40 years ago, 80 percent of adults in this country were permanently immune to diphtheria because of having had a clinical or subclinical form during childhood. This situation is no longer true. Consequently, adults should receive booster shots of diphtheria toxoid every ten years. Serious reactions to diphtheria toxoid (a dead vaccine) are rare.

Tetanus. Cases of tetanus also occur every year. Although the toxoid vaccine is thoroughly safe and effective, its protection wanes over the years, and booster shots are required. There is lack of agreement on how frequently boosters should be given. The American Academy of Pediatrics officially says every ten years past the ages of four to six. The American College of Surgeons believes boosters are necessary every five years for minor wounds of the sort that are not seen and treated by a doctor. (Even adults should have routine tetanus boosters at least every ten years.)

Whooping Cough. This is the most uncertain of the three components of DTP vaccine. It does not always result in complete immunity. Rare instances of permanent brain damage have followed its use, although in some of these cases the injuries were due to faulty administration. It is prone to cause brief reactions with fever. For these reasons, boosters are not recommended routinely past the age of four to six years, when the dangers of whooping cough are judged less serious than the dangers of the vaccine. In England, serious reactions to this vaccine have been frequent enough so that its use has been temporarily abandoned. However, the mortality rate among infants with whooping cough under age one and the complication rate among older children are high enough to exceed by far the minimal risk of the vaccine.

Polio

Infants should receive two or three doses of the live vaccine (Sabin, containing types 1, 2, and 3) orally, starting at two months with the second and third doses following, separated by one or two months. A booster series should be given at one and one-half to two years and at four to six years. Children not immunized during infancy should receive a total of three or four doses depending upon their age.

There are still outbreaks of paralytic polio in this country, and there is no doubt of the safety of the Sabin vaccine for children. If

adults who are not immune travel to countries where polio is still uncontrolled, they should receive immunization. Current thinking is that they need not be if they are not exposed by foreign travel because the risk of exposure in this country is minimal. We disagree. Too many cases of polio have occurred in persons 30 years of age and older. Sabin vaccine carries a small risk for adults but the dead Salk vaccine does not. Adults who are not immune should receive an initial series of Salk vaccine (which confers temporary immunity) followed by a full series of Sabin vaccine for permanent protection.

Measles, Mumps, Rubella

The live, triple vaccine, MMR, should be given to all children at 15 months. It confers long term and probably lifelong immunity against all three diseases.

Measles. Among the common childhood contagious diseases, this one threatens with serious complications. Encephalitis occurs in one of every one thousand cases of natural measles. The risk of encephalitis from the vaccine is less than one in one million, and the disease complications of pneumonia and ear infections are never seen with immunization.

Rubella and Mumps. These diseases are relatively mild in children but the first can be devastating to the unborn child, and the second can be complicated with encephalitis and deafness. The vaccines are harmless to children (except for rare, transient arthritis in older children from rubella vaccine).

Smallpox

Vaccination against smallpox is no longer practiced in the United States. The risk of the live vaccine, although minimal, is still in excess of the risk of contracting smallpox, which is nil. It is anticipated that smallpox will be eradicated from the entire world in the near future.

Other Vaccines

Vaccines against typhoid, typhus, yellow fever, influenza, Rocky Mountain spotted fever, meningococci, and pneumococci are presently available. None of these is yet recommended for children except in instances when the child will be at special risk. Consult your doctor if you are in doubt.

Related Topics: Diphtheria, Encephalitis, Measles, Mumps, Pneumonia, Polio, Rubella, Tetanus, Whooping Cough

MEDICATIONS

When a proper diagnosis has been made and the most appropriate medicine selected, the child's physician is home free. But the third, and often most decisive factor, is the parent's responsibility to administer the medicine correctly. Ten to thirty percent of treatment failures are directly due to inadequate administration of an effective drug. If the doctor's directions are vague, or you don't understand them, ask for clarification.

Dosage

Most medications are prescribed in proportion to a child's weight. Accurate liquid measurements are important. "One teaspoonful" does not mean any old teaspoon. It means one measuring teaspoonful, or 5.0 cubic-centimeters (cc). "One-half teaspoonful" does not mean guessing when an ordinary spoon is half full. It means 2.5 cc, or a full half-teaspoon measuring spoon. (Of course, after you have measured the medicine you may transfer the potion to any convenient spoon for giving the medicine to your child.) If your child vomits within one hour of receiving medication you can assume that the dose has been lost and repeat it.

Timing

"Four times a day" means that four doses should be given within every 24 hours, but the

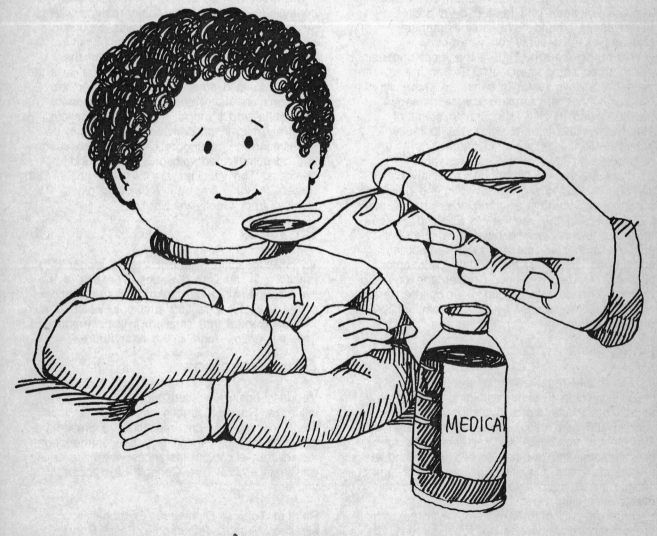

With the right approach you can easily get your child to take his medicine.

child's sleep doesn't need to be interrupted. Common sense dictates that the four doses should be spread out as widely as is possible and convenient while the child is awake. "Every six hours" means just that: one dose is given every six hours around the clock.

Duration

Most relapses and many complications are the result of stopping medication prematurely. Often a child feels and acts well before he is well. Earaches stop, fevers vanish, coughs subside, and appetites return when germs are merely stunned and healing scarcely begun. Strep infections require 10 or more days of antibiotic therapy before the infection is gone. Urinary tract infections and ear infections often take even longer to cure, although symptoms may disappear in a day. So be sure you continue any medication for as long as it has been prescribed. "Give for 10 full days," "Continue for two weeks," "Give until finished," are not suggestions, but directions with a purpose. They should be considered orders.

Methods

Administration of medicines to children is a vital skill for all responsible parents to master. Of course, infants and children are not always willing and eager to take their medicines. On the other hand, since you know what's best for your child, you are the one to decide. A parent who reports to a doctor that a child will not accept a medicine forces the doctor to resort to a second-best treatment and sometimes to hospitalize the child for nurses to administer the medication.

Infants and Toddlers

Oral, liquid medicines can be given to young children directly from a spoon (after careful measuring) or by a non glass medicine dropper used to squirt the liquid slowly into a cheek. Take care to avoid directing the stream forcefully against the back of the throat and down the windpipe. Disguising medicine in a small quantity of juice, ice cream, applesauce, and the like is acceptable, provided the child takes the entire potion. A sweet treat may be offered after medication to cut the objectionable taste.

A young child, approached reassuringly, kindly, but firmly, often will passively accept medication. If the child struggles and refuses,

other approaches must be found to administer the medicine. An enraged or terrified child can be soothed into cooperation by being totally immobilized. This is accomplished by "mummying." With the arms pinioned to the sides, the child is wrapped tightly in a folded sheet from neck to toes. Within minutes a mummied and cuddled child will be ready to accept oral medicines, at least on the second or third try. Any attempt to spit out the medicine should be countered by a restraining hand placed calmly over the mouth. (Swaddling or mummying is equally effective for administering nose drops.)

Although some infants and toddlers accept chewable tablets of medicine or even swallow whole tablets or capsules, these forms of medication are dangerous in this age group. A child under three can easily choke to death on a bulky pill. If liquid forms of the medicine are not available, tablets should be mashed and the contents of capsules emptied into juice or food before administering them to a toddler.

Older Children

Many children over five or six can swallow tablets and capsules whole. Start with relatively unimportant medicines such as aspirin when your child has a headache. And only attempt it if he is willing. Help him to learn to swallow a pill by placing it on the back of his tongue before giving him something to drink, or include it in a half-teaspoonful of applesauce, jelly, or ice cream and have him swallow the entire thing. (A special glass that delivers a pill into the mouth automatically when the first gulp of the liquid in the glass is taken is also available.)

Rectal Medications

Many medicines are available in suppository form. They include antiemetics, aspirin, acetaminophen, antihistamines, sedatives, anticonvulsants, antibiotics, antiasthmatics, cough medicines, and laxatives. Although valuable when a child is vomiting or unconscious, they are not as well absorbed as oral medications and have limited applicability. **Caution:** They are not to be used routinely as a substitute on a child who is reluctant to accept oral medicines. Teaching the child the necessity of cooperating is also an important issue.

(Those medicines referred to under each ailment profile as "OTC" are over-the-counter preparations and may be obtained without a prescription.)

LYMPH NODES—INFECTION FIGHTERS

Lymph nodes are sometimes referred to as lymph glands, although they are not true glands. In their usual state, they are an eighth- to a quarter-inch in size and are widely distributed throughout the body. Ordinarily, they feel like B-B shot lying just beneath the skin. Attached neither to the skin nor to the underlying tissues, lymph nodes are "poppable," that is, they can be easily moved a short distance parallel to the skin by an exploring finger. This characteristic readily distinguishes them from cysts, which are usually attached to the skin, and from deeper structures which cannot be moved.

The following are the most important lymph node sites:

- quarter-inch in front of the ears (preauricular nodes);
- quarter-inch to a half-inch behind the ears (postauricular);
- at the base of the skull on both sides (occipital);
- under the angle of the jaw, and extending like a string of beads down the sides of the neck in front of the strap muscles (anterior cervical nodes);
- a similar string just behind the same strap muscle (posterior cervical);
- in the midline under the chin (submental);
- in the armpits (axillary);
- in the folds of the elbows (epitrochlear);
- above the crease in the groin (inguinal); and
- below the crease in the groin (femoral).

Lymph nodes are also found within the chest and abdomen but cannot be felt on examination.

All lymph nodes are situated along thin-walled tubes called lymphatic vessels, which resemble and roughly follow the course of the veins in the body. They do not contain blood, however, but a thin, clear, slightly sticky liquid called lymph, which resembles the clear, watery fluid that oozes from a superficial scrape or that forms within a blister caused by rubbing. The appearance of red streaks is typical of impending blood poisoning and is caused by infection rising along the lymphatic vessels.

Function

Lymph nodes are composed of closely packed congregations of cells called lymphocytes, which are also found in the circulating blood. Lymphocytes manufacture various types of antibodies, substances that fight disease, cause allergic reactions, and reject foreign organic material. Lymph nodes also trap microorganisms that penetrate the skin or mucous membranes and prevent them from spreading throughout the body. Some germs prove too much for the lymph nodes to handle, however, and a node itself may become infected. When this happens, the node enlarges and becomes more tender; the overlying skin becomes red. If the node is killed by the infection, it breaks down into pus, which may erupt through the skin as would a deep-seated boil. It is no longer "poppable" under the skin, but becomes anchored to the skin or to deeper tissues.

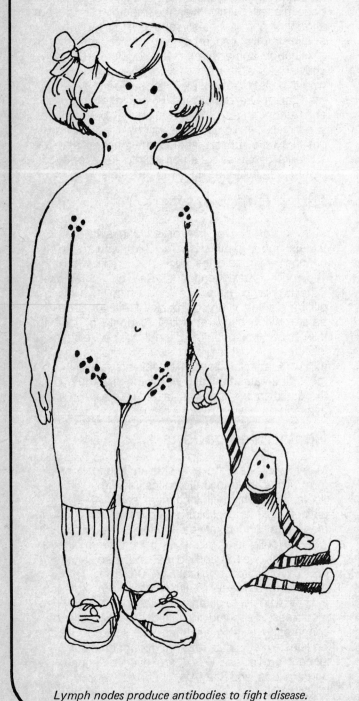

Lymph nodes produce antibodies to fight disease.

LYMPH NODES—INFECTION FIGHTERS

Diagnostic Significance

Ordinarily lymph nodes are not tender unless they are squeezed or unless they are infected. When infected, the lymph nodes swell to several sizes larger than normal and become mildly tender. Only those nodes swell when the area of the body they guard is threatened by infection. An insect bite, a boil, impetigo, an infected scratch, chicken pox, burns, splinters, or any other lesion may cause swelling.

Lesions of the upper face or front of the scalp affect the preauricular glands on that side of the back of the scalp, the postauricular, and occipital glands. Lesions of the lower face or teeth may cause the submental glands to swell. Infections of the throat, tonsils, or back teeth affect the anterior and sometimes the posterior cervical nodes. The epitrochlear glands respond to lesions of the fingers, hands, and forearm, and the axillary glands guard the same areas, plus the upper arm, armpit, and side of the chest. The inguinal and femoral glands swell from problems of the toes, foot, leg, arms, and genitalia. These regional responses of the nodes allow you to pinpoint the area in which to search for trouble.

Generalized infections may involve all the lymph nodes. Commonest of these diseases is infectious mononucleosis which involves all the lymphoid tissue of the body. Since the spleen, tonsils, and adenoids are also lymphoid tissue, they also become enlarged. The spleen is an organ the size of half an orange located under the left lower lateral ribs. (Composed mostly of lymphocytes, it is connected to blood vessels instead of to lymphatic vessels, however.) Other generalized diseases, including chicken pox and leukemia (cancer of the white blood cells), also produce overall lymph node enlargement.

Rubella is the only common illness that results in swelling of the preauricular, postauricular, and occipital lymph nodes to the exclusion of the other nodes. This is a diagnostic clue in the presence of a generalized rash.

When your child is ill, note which, if any, lymph nodes are swollen. If they are mildly swollen, that indicates they are doing their job. If they are greatly enlarged (compare with healthy node size), too tender, adherent to the skin, and red, the illness requires help from your physician.

Related Topics: Blood Poisoning; Burns; Chicken Pox; Cuts; Glands, Swollen; Impetigo; Infectious Mononucleosis; Insect Bites; Leukemia; Rubella; Scrapes

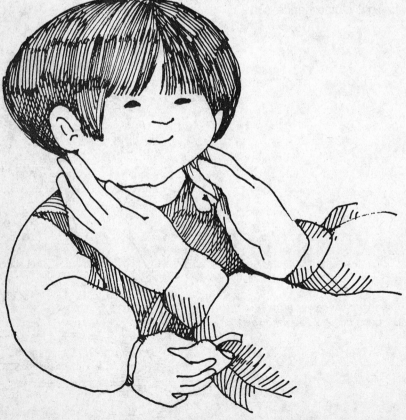

Infected lymph nodes are swollen and tender.

ACNE

Description

Commonly occurring during adolescence, acne is a condition of the skin, particularly of the face, but also is seen on the chest and back. In its mildest form, acne appears as large blackheads and whiteheads (blind blackheads). The formation of "zits," which look like infected pimples, is a more severe case. The worst cases form cysts and scars.

Believed for generations to be related to a lack of cleanliness and to a diet of junk foods, acne is now attributed to hormonal action, and the normal processes of change during the adolescent years. Zits are the result of normal skin germs breaking down the oil in the blackheads and forming irritating substances. The pus that results is not an infection.

Diagnosis

The skin breaks out in tiny, red bumps which may or may not be open. Lumps under the skin indicate that the acne has become cystic.

Home Treatment

Wash the affected area with mild soap twice a day. Apply acne preparations containing sulfur, resorcin, salicylic acid, or mild benzoyl peroxide after washing. Large, unsightly blackheads can be gently removed with a blackhead spoon, available at your pharmacy. A restriction of the teenager's diet is unnecessary.

Precautions

● To avoid making a case of acne worse, adolescents should stay away from skin irritants such as motor oil, gasoline and oil-containing cosmetics. ● Do not squeeze or pick zits as scarring may result. Do not treat acne in infants. ● And if acne does not improve or if cysts develop, see your doctor.

Doctor's Treatment

Acne treatment has vastly improved in the past five years. Doctors now prescribe new vitamin A ointment or liquid or prescription-strength benzoyl peroxide for local application. Long-term oral therapy using tetracycline or other antibiotics is safe and effective. The local application of antibiotics is still experimental, but promising. Cysts may be injected with tiny doses of steroids, and disfiguring scars can be removed by a dermatologist or plastic surgeon without hospitalization once the acne is under control. (**Never allow x-ray treatment of acne.**)

To zap acne have your growing child wash twice daily with a mild soap.

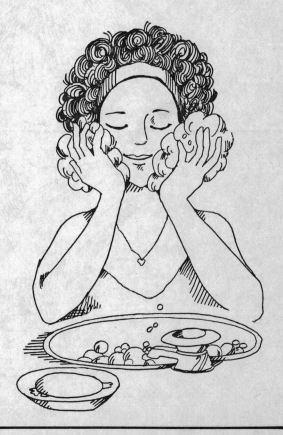

Description

Anemia exists when there is too little hemoglobin in the blood. Hemoglobin is the substance that carries oxygen in the blood and gives it its red color. Normally, hemoglobin is contained within the red blood cells (RBCs). A child can be anemic because there are too few RBCs, because each RBC contains too little hemoglobin, or as a result of both conditions.

There are more than thirty types of anemia, each with its own cause and treatment. The most common is iron deficiency anemia. Anemia can occur at any age. Some forms run in families; other are acquired.

Among the commonest causes of anemia are: the loss of blood by internal or external bleeding; a poor diet with inadequate intake of the nutrients needed to manufacture hemoglobin (iron, protein, folic acid, vitamin B_{12}, and copper); a failure to absorb the nutrients, even though they are eaten; the formation of abnormal (short-lived) RBCs; an inability of the bone marrow to produce RBCs fast enough; and the too-rapid destruction of normal RBCs within the body. In addition to the many diseases that are forms of anemia, many other illnesses can produce anemia.

Diagnosis

Periodic examinations and a history taken by a doctor can help catch anemia early, an important factor in treatment. Although most cases of anemia produce no symptoms, tiredness, shortness of breath, rapid pulse, and jaundice may be clues. If a child looks pale, check the nailbeds, the inside of the eyelids, and the membranes of the mouth for additional colorlessness. Also, be vigilant for: vomiting of blood or blood in the stools (red or tarry-black bowel movements); excessive menstruation; a grossly inadequate diet; chronic diarrhea with loss of ingested foods; and exposure to poisonous substances. The presence and type of anemia can only be determined by laboratory tests. If one family member has anemia, watch for symptoms in others.

Home Treatment

Never attempt to treat anemia yourself. The wrong treatment can be harmful and will make a proper medical diagnosis difficult. All children should receive a balanced diet to prevent nutritionally caused anemia.

Precautions

● Iron overdosing is the second commonest poisoning among children in this country. If supplemental iron is prescribed by your doctor, keep it out of the reach of children. Some iron medicines are sweet and mistaken for candy.

Doctor's Treatment

The testing for anemia is extensive. In addition to giving your child a physical examination, taking a history and simple total blood count, your doctor is likely to take a reticulocyte (young RBC) count, platelet count, measurement of iron and of the iron-binding capacity in the blood, hemoglobin electrophoretic pattern, sickle cell test, urinalysis, test of stools for hidden blood, examination of bone marrow, test for poisons, examination of the child's parents' blood, X ray of the intestinal tract, and blood chemistries among others.

Once anemia is confirmed, your doctor will run additional blood tests to determine the type. The treatment prescribed may include adding supplemental iron and vitamins to the diet, a change in diet, and—though rarely—a blood transfusion. Iron or vitamin injections also are rarely called for and, if given, are administered for the first one or two doses only.

As treatment proceeds, be sure additional tests are scheduled to check on the effectiveness of the treatment. The proof of proper treatment is in the cure.

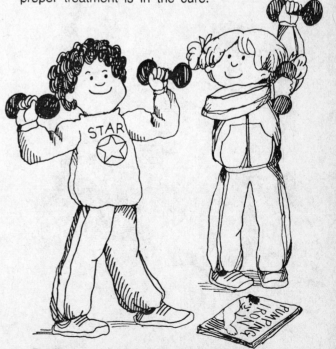

Feeding your child the right foods will help prevent iron deficiency anemia.

ANIMAL BITES

Description

Animal bites that break the skin are cuts, puncture wounds, or scrapes and should be treated as such. But animal bites have other special characteristics: they are prone to infection because of bacteria in the animal's mouth, and they may cause lockjaw (tetanus) or rabies.

Rabies is a fatal disease of the central nervous system to which all mammals are susceptible. It is caused by a virus that can be seen microscopically and identified within the brain of affected animals. Transmitted through the saliva of the sick animal, rabies is most commonly found in the United States among skunks, foxes, cattle, dogs, bats, cats, and raccoons. It is rare among squirrels, chipmunks, rats, and mice. There is no risk from caged, domestic pets such as gerbils, guinea pigs, hamsters, and white mice.

Diagnosis

Bites are usually obvious from their appearance and from the child's telling of the tale. Claw wounds may be indistinguishable from bites but are treated in the same way because of possible contamination by the animal's saliva. Bruises without a break in the skin are not a threat of rabies, and are handled like any other bruises.

Home Treatment

Wash the wound with soap and water and flush with water. Apply antiseptic to minor wounds. If a wild animal did the biting, catch and hold it if this can be done without endangering anyone else; otherwise, kill and preserve it for inspection of its brain for rabies. If it's a domestic animal, catch and impound or kill and preserve it. Find out if the domestic animal was vaccinated against rabies and determine the child's tetanus toxoid status. Report the wound to your doctor immediately for advice concerning rabies, tetanus, and repair of the wound. In some states animal bites must be reported to the police.

Precautions

- Keep children current on tetanus boosters.
- Always contact your doctor about treatment in the case of animal bites.

Doctor's Treatment

Because of the high incidence of infection your doctor may elect not to suture wounds. If cosmetic consideration necessitates closure, treatment first includes removal of the injured tissue and a thorough cleansing. Oral antibiotics may be prescribed. Also, your doctor will give a tetanus booster or human antitoxin to the patient if needed.

The decision whether or not to give antirabies vaccine, with or without antiserum, is complex. There's a good possibility of serious reactions. Your doctor will arrange for examination of the animal for the presence of rabies. A pet properly immunized against rabies can still transmit rabies, although this possibility is minimal. If the animal is not caught, the decision depends upon prevalence of rabies in your area, circumstances of the bite (provoked or unprovoked), and the species of the animal. Local health departments can provide information to help you make this decision. If you're still in doubt contact the Center for Disease Control, Rabies Investigations Unit, Atlanta, Georgia. Call for consultation, 8:00 a.m. to 5:00 p.m. E.S.T.—(404) 633-3311; off-duty hours, call (404) 633-2176

Related Topics: Cat Scratch Fever, Cuts, Bruises, Puncture Wounds, Scrapes, Tetanus

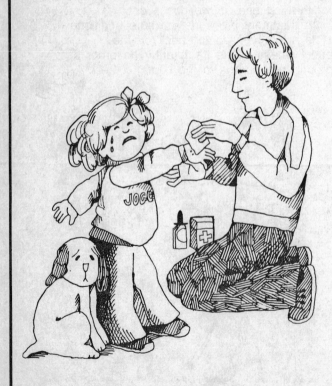

Have your pets immunized against rabies.

APPENDICITIS

Description

Appendicitis is an infection (inflammation) of the appendix. The appendix is a hollow tube about the size of your little finger that forms a blind pouch at the site where the small intestine joins the large intestine. In 99 percent of all children the appendix lies in the lower right quarter of the child's abdomen. Appendicitis can occur at any age. If not surgically removed the infection worsens until the appendix bursts, and the infection spreads rapidly throughout the abdomen. An infected appendix may perforate (rupture) within hours of the initial pain or not for a day or two.

Diagnosis

Any abdominal pain in your child is due to appendicitis until proven otherwise. Typically, the pain of appendicitis is constant; it does not come and go as do cramps. Once it starts, it grows worse by the hour. The pain may start in the pit of the stomach, but it soon moves to the right, lower quarter of the abdomen. The pain is made worse by walking or just moving about. The abdomen is tender to a gentle pressure in the right, lower quadrant, more tender than in other areas. There may be nausea and vomiting, but these symptoms usually start only after the pain has started.

Generally, there is a low-grade fever (100°F, oral; 101°F, rectal), but the temperature may range anywhere from normal to 104°F. Bowel movements are usually normal, but there may be diarrhea. Urination may be painful. Diagnosis is difficult because all of these signs may not be present.

Home Treatment

Try applying gentle heat, as with a heating pad turned to "low." If pain gets worse it is probably appendicitis. **Never apply cold;** this can mask symptoms of appendicitis. Try Dramamine, or Emetrol antinauseants; again, if your child gets worse instead of better there is a strong possibility of appendicitis. Do not give pain killers such as paregoric or codeine. Aspirin and acetaminophen are safe but useless. Allow only clear liquids by mouth. **Never give a laxative or enema.**

Always suspect appendicitis when your child complains of a stomach ache.

Precautions

● If pain persists in the lower, right quadrant of the abdomen for more than two hours, despite home treatment measures, call your doctor.

Doctor's Treatment

Because the only acceptable treatment for appendicitis is surgical removal of the appendix (an appendectomy), your doctor must be reasonably sure of the diagnosis. In addition to the abdomen, your child's chest and throat will be examined because a throat infection and pneumonia can mimic symptoms of appendicitis. A rectal examination will also be performed and a blood count and a urinalysis done. (These last two tests do not prove or disprove appendicitis, however.) An X ray may be called for.

Once tests are complete, your doctor may decide to operate or to admit your child to a hospital to watch him for a few hours until the diagnosis becomes more certain. Unjustified surgery is to be avoided, but the rule of safety is to operate on a child who may have appendicitis rather than postpone surgery until the appendix ruptures.

Related Topics: Stomach Ache, Acute; Stomach Ache, Chronic

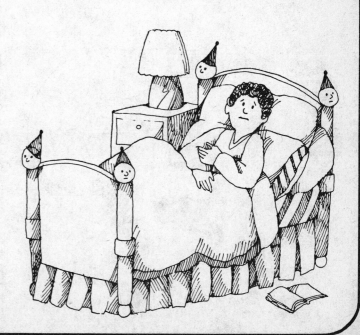

25

ARTHRITIS

Description

Arthritis is an inflammation of any joint or joints, including those of the fingers, toes, wrists, ankles, elbows, knees, shoulders, hips, jaw, and spine. Five types are common to childhood: rheumatoid arthritis; acute rheumatic fever; infectious arthritis; allergic arthritis; and arthritis of rubella.

Rheumatoid arthritis can occur at any age past one year old. So far the cause is unknown. It may involve one or several joints which become swollen, warm, stiff, and mildly to moderately painful, but not usually red. The neck is involved in 50 percent of the cases. Arthritis may appear months before or after other signs of illness, such as fever, irritability, loss of appetite, and a fine, pink rash.

Arthritis associated with *acute rheumatic fever* usually involves many joints which become red, swollen, and extremely tender. Evidence of generalized illness is also present.

Infectious (purulent) *arthritis* is an inflammation within a joint caused by various bacterial diseases including staphylococcal, streptococcal, pneumococcal, and salmonella infections. This type of arthritis most often occurs in infants less than one year old. In older children and adults it can be the result of puncture wounds near the joints. In this type of arthritis, the joint is severely tender, swollen, and red; fever is usually present.

In *allergic arthritis* the joints are stiff, swollen, and red, but pain is minimal. The disease is caused by an allergic reaction to insect stings, medications, foods, or inhalants. It is generally accompanied by hives.

Arthritis of rubella is a benign, self-curing arthritis, which occurs as a complication of rubella (German measles) or as a reaction to rubella vaccine, especially in older children.

Diagnosis

Arthritis isn't confined to the elderly. It also occurs in children of all ages. Arthritis should be considered whenever there is pain and a limited ability to move any joint, unless there has been a documented injury. Determining the type of arthritis is best left up to the doctor.

Home Treatment

No home treatment is safe until a correct diagnosis has been made as it may delay and obscure proper diagnosis. If your doctor is not immediately available, pain relievers containing aspirin, acetaminophen, or codeine will temporarily reduce the discomfort. Rest or immobilize the affected joints. If arthritis is thought to be from an allergy, relief can be obtained by using oral antihistamines.

Precautions

● Infectious arthritis is an acute emergency, and delay of treatment for 24 hours may result in permanent damage to a joint. Rheumatoid arthritis and rheumatic fever require prompt treatment to minimize damage but are not considered emergencies. ● Consider rheumatoid arthritis if the child has a prolonged obscure fever, particularly if there is stiffness of the joints and neck, even when external signs of arthritis (redness, tenderness, swelling) are absent.

Doctor's Treatment

Unless the disease is obviously allergic arthritis or arthritis from rubella, multiple tests are required. These tests may include: X rays, a wide variety of blood tests; blood culture; aspiration of fluid from the joint for testing; electrocardiogram; and a stool culture. Treatment may include antibiotic therapy, drainage of the joints, prolonged administration of large doses of aspirin (aspirin substitutes do not have the same effect); or oral steroids. If large doses of aspirin are prescribed, aspirin blood levels should be tested regularly.

Related Topics: Growing Pains, Hip Problems, Knee Pains, Puncture Wounds, Sprains & Dislocations

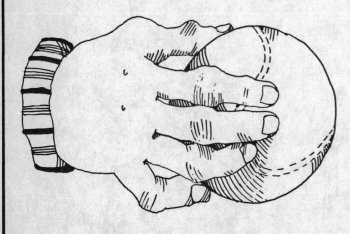

Arthritis is treatable, but it's up to your doctor to diagnose it first.

Description

Asthma is an allergic reaction of the bronchial tree. It is a major and potentially dangerous form of allergy characterized by spasms of the smooth muscles of the bronchial tubes and the accumulation of thick mucus within these tubes. Shortness of breath, cough, sensations of air hunger, and wheezing are symptomatic, and it becomes harder for the child to breathe out than to breathe in. Wheezing is a high-pitched whistling sound more prominent on exhalation than on inhalation (in contrast to croup).

Asthma is caused by an allergy to inhalants (animal dander, pollens, dust, feathers, molds), and less commonly to foods, medicines, and insect stings. Attacks may be triggered by physical exertion, upper respiratory infections, emotions, or irritants such as smoke or chlorine. Fever is absent unless it is caused by a concurrent infection. The tendency to have allergies (including asthma) runs in families.

Diagnosis

The characteristic sound of wheezing is an asthma "give-away." The disease can be confirmed by rapid response to antiallergic medications. Asthma in a child under two is difficult to diagnose. History may be helpful especially if an asthma attack coincides with exposure to a cat, dog, horse, or other animal with hair or fur; is seasonal, as during tree, grass, or ragweed pollination; or occurs at night when the child is sleeping on a feather pillow.

Home Treatment

No home treatment is recommended for the first attack; your doctor will confirm diagnosis and select a specific treatment. In an emergency antihistamines may be given by mouth (in proper dose for weight) to allay the attack, but the treatment isn't reliably effective.

After the diagnosis is established, home treatment is important and effective. Prescribed medications should be administered promptly at onset of an attack; they are less effective after attack is under way. Rid your home of the identified causes of asthma allergy—pets, feather pillows and comforters, house dust, and sources of mold. Avoid exposing your child to such airborn irritants as insecticides, smoke and paint fumes.

Precautions

● Do not use aerosol antiasthma medications on children. They can be dangerous and make

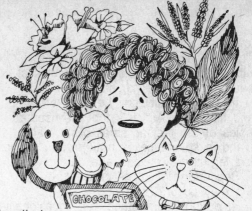

Not all wheezes are caused by asthma. Check with your doctor.

other medications less effective. ● Do not use rectally administered aminophylline or theophylline if avoidable; this route is unreliable and may result in the administration of improper dosage (either too little or too much). ● Do not let an attack go untreated. Improperly treated, frequent attacks of asthma can result in permanent damage to the lungs and bronchial tubes. ● Because not all wheezes are asthma, have your doctor check your suspicions.

Doctor's Treatment

Your doctor will initiate treatment by taking a complete and detailed history, conducting a physical examination (perhaps including an X ray) and running a series of five to twenty skin tests of suspected materials to which the child may be allergic. The substances identified as causes must be eliminated from the child's environment wherever possible. Diagnosis can be confirmed by response to medication.

Oral medications for use during an attack may include theophylline, aminophylline, ephedrine, metaproterenol, potassium iodide, antihistamines, and steroids. The same drugs may be recommended for daily use to prevent attacks. The newest medicines that can be used daily for prevention are cromolyn sodium and beclomethasone by inhalation. Children also may be desensitized to causative substances by weekly to monthly injections of increasing amounts of the irritating substances over a period of one to ten years. Severe attacks may require hospitalization for intravenous medications and fluids and for oxygen.

The treatment for asthma should produce good results. If the attacks do not lessen within one to three months, discuss a new approach with your doctor or ask for a second opinion.

Related Topics: Bronchiolitis, Bronchitis, Conjunctivitis, Croup, Hay Fever, Hives

ATHLETE'S FOOT

Description

Athlete's foot is an infection of the skin of the feet by one of several funguses that grow best in the presence of moisture. The mildest cases cause itching, scaling, and cracking between the toes, particularly between the fourth and fifth toes. Athlete's foot may spread to the soles of the feet as small blisters and scaling, and in severe cases may spread to the ankle and leg. It may invade and deform the toenails. Secondary infections caused by scratching may occur. The disease is commonest during adolescence, but occasionally it appears in infants.

Diagnosis

Tentative diagnosis is based on the scaling and cracking appearance of the feet and the itching that accompanies it.

Home Treatment

Apply fungicidal ointment such as Whitfields ointment once or twice a day (half strength for delicate skin), or use OTC ointments containing undecylenic acid, tolnaftate, or undecylenate.

Caution: Many "incurable" cases of athlete's foot are not athlete's foot but are rashes from contact dermatitis caused by the treatment. Rubber-soled or plastic-soled shoes should be avoided for routine use to minimize sweating. Use cotton socks for absorption, preferably white to avoid contact dermatitis from dyes.

Precautions

● Continue treatment until skin is completely clear; funguses not completely treated flare up.
● If improvement is not prompt and lasting see your doctor; your diagnosis may be wrong. ●
Many OTC medications for athlete's foot can cause contact dermatitis in susceptible people.

Doctor's Treatment

Diagnosis is confirmed by scraping the skin and culturing the fungus or identifying it under a microscope. Your doctor may prescribe other fungicidal ointments or lotions or an oral fungicide. If a secondary infection is present your doctor may prescribe oral antibiotics and soaking in a solution of potassium permanganate or aluminum sulfate and calcium acetate.

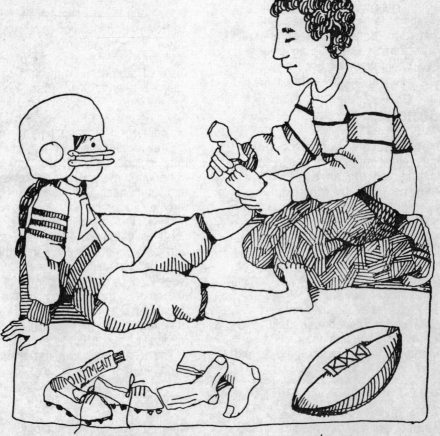

Use fungicidal ointment at the first sign of athlete's foot.

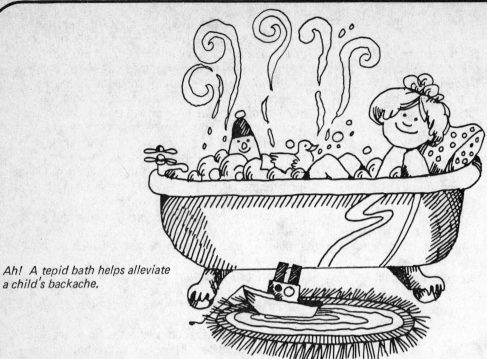

Ah! A tepid bath helps alleviate a child's backache.

Description

Soreness and backache are almost as common in children as in adults. Almost as soon as children are old enough to complain of pain and to locate it, they experience occasional backaches. Frequency increases through adolescence. Most pains are the result of strenuous activities that cause stress to the muscles and ligaments of the back. These back problems are limited and self-curing. More serious back pain may be caused by infections and abnormalities of the kidneys, malformations and abnormal curvatures of the spine, a defect of the growth plates of the vertebrae (Scheuermann's disease), compression fractures, and arthritis.

Diagnosis

Backache caused by stress produces pain and slight tenderness in the muscles that run up and down either side of the midline of the back. Pain is aggravated by bending and twisting and is lessened by rest, aspirin, and mild heat. If physical activity is curtailed the condition improves slowly day by day.

Backache of renal (kidney) origin is apt to be one-sided and may be accompanied by urinary symptoms such as burning on urination, frequency, and discoloration of the urine. Backache that is limited to one spot in the midline or to an extended length of the midline may be a sprain or may even be a symptom of a disease of the vertebrae. Abnormal curves of the spine can often be seen. Minor curves

to one side or the other can best be seen with the child undressed and bending forward to touch the floor with both hands; even a slight curve (scoliosis) causes the back to appear asymmetrical in this position.

Home Treatment

If there is no visible deformity, no fever, and no localization of the pain, treatment with aspirin or acetaminophen, mild heat from an electric pad or a tepid bath, and bed rest are safe. If the mattress is not extra firm, a bedboard under the mattress (a piece of plywood will do) helps relieve the discomfort. Have your child avoid any strenuous physical activity until the pain has been absent at least a week.

Precautions

● If fever, urinary symptoms, severe pain, or sharply localized pain is present see your doctor. ● Do not use muscle relaxant medications on children without your doctor's approval.

Doctor's Treatment

In addition to a careful history and physical examination, urinalysis, X rays, blood count, and sedimentation rate may be required. Specific treatment depends upon the discovered cause, and may well be the same as home treatment. Therapy might also include antibiotics, orthopedic exercises, back brace, or even hospitalization and traction.

BALDNESS

Description

Baldness is a loss of hair which may be local or general. Some infants are born bald or nearly so and develop a full head of hair during their first two years. Rarely do babies remain bald for life (a form of congenital baldness). Some babies are born with a full head of hair. They may remain that way or their original hair may be replaced by a second and permanent growth. Rarely is hair lost during infancy and never replaced (another form of congenital baldness).

Infants commonly rub off a band of hair in the back against the crib or playpen mat. Their hair will grow back. Drawing the hair tightly into pigtails, braids, or ponytails also may result in temporary bald spots. Children with the habit of twisting and playing with strands of hair may produce the same results. Emotionally disturbed children may pull out their hair by the handfuls (trichotillomania). This condition requires more treatment of what's going on in the mind than a concern with the migrating bald spots.

Alopecia areata is a condition which results in the sudden appearance of round or oval areas that are totally bare. The bald scalp is completely normal in appearance or slightly pink. Although temporary, the condition may last for months or years. Rarely is the entire head involved. The cause is unknown.

Ringworm of the scalp produces scattered bald spots. The scalp is scaly, and the bald spots are studded with broken-off stubble of hair.

Hereditary baldness is confined to males and causes baldness at the temples or the top of the scalp. Occasionally this type of baldness starts during adolescence.

Teenagers often complain that they are "going bald" when they see loose hair after combing. This condition is merely a thinning of the hair, and is normal and non-progressive.

Malfunction of the parathyroid glands (hyperparathyroidism) may result in scattered baldness. The disease is accompanied by other signs of illness.

Impetigo and other infections of the scalp produce temporary bald spots.

Diagnosis

Inspect the scalp closely for evidence of ringworm or infection and for the presence of broken and regrowing hairs. Diagnosis also depends upon history and observation of habits.

Home Treatment

Alopecia areata is treated with patience and time; hereditary and congenital baldness with understanding, love, and a hairpiece.

Precautions

● Do not treat baldness with OTC preparations.
● Do not consult cosmetologists. See a qualified dermatologist.

Doctor's Treatment

Alopecia areata is sometimes successfully treated with steroids either applied or locally injected. Hyperparathyrodism must be diagnosed by blood tests and treated with large doses of vitamin D and special diet.

Baldness in a baby is common and has many causes.

Related Topics: Impetigo, Ringworm

Description

Many children cannot remain dry through the night before they are four or five. About ten percent of all children over the age of five are bedwetters. Children of any age may have occasional accidents at night, especially if ill or in exhausted sleep—conditions that do not represent true bedwetting (enuresis). Five to ten percent of children who bedwet have a physical disease such as an infection or abnormality of the urinary tract, diabetes, or neurological disorder. If a child wets himself both day and night a physical disease is likely. Disease is also probable if enuresis develops a year or more after night training has been established. All other cases are considered functional; that is, no identifiable organ disorder is indicated as its cause. Some cases seem to be hereditary, with siblings and parents also having been bedwetters. Some are caused by overemphasis by the family on toilet training, others by taking children out of their night diapers too soon or by waking children to urinate in an effort to night-train. Some children have emotional problems which manifest themselves in bedwetting. Still, the cause of many cases of bedwetting remains unknown.

Diagnosis

A child who consistently wets the bed after age five has enuresis.

Home Treatment

Before any home treatment of chronic bedwetting can proceed, a complete urinalysis and urine culture should be done to rule out urinary tract infection and diabetes. Then, the best treatment is avoidance. **Do not** take a child out of night diapers until he consistently remains dry. **Do not** make a big fuss about daytime training. **Do not** try to shame a child into remaining dry at night. Withholding liquids during late afternoon and evening hours may be construed as cruel and undeserved punishment. Behavior modification techniques with reward for success and neutral reaction toward failure, rarely work. Devices called enuratones, which awaken the child as urination starts, have been successful with older children but are not universally approved of by psychiatrists. Rubber sheets, draw sheets, and soakers are helpful until enuresis is corrected.

Precautions

● Do not let a minor problem like enuresis become a major destructive factor in your relationship with your child. Anger and hate between parent and child are more costly than an extra wash. ● Do not allow siblings to taunt a bedwetter.

Doctor's Treatment

Your doctor will insist first upon conducting a physical examination and urinalysis. The doctor may suggest: X rays of the urinary tract or consultation with a urologist; imipramine (an antidepressant) by mouth at bedtime for a trial period; dextroamphetamine, dilantin, or caffeine also on a temporary basis; or a program of behavior modification. All may be worth a try. There has been reported success with a special external catheter into which the penis is inserted at night.

Related Topics: Diabetes, Urinary Tract Infection

Rule out disease and treat bedwetting with patience.

BIRTHMARKS

Description

Almost 50 percent of infants are born with red or salmon-colored marks on the midforehead, upper eyelids, upper lip ("angels' kisses") or on the back of the scalp and neck ("stork bites"). These marks, which are sometimes quite extensive, fade and disappear during the first years of life.

Many black, Oriental, and Caucasian babies who are destined to become brunettes have smooth, blue-back marks on their backs and buttocks. Called "mongolian spots," these birthmarks are often mistaken for large bruises. They gradually disappear and, with rare exception, are gone by adolescence.

One in ten babies develops one or more strawberry marks during the first month of life. These are usually not apparent at birth or are visible as slightly pale spots on the skin. As the child grows, the marks become brilliant red, are often raised, and vary in diameter from one-quarter inch to two inches. They appear on any part of the body and increase in size for weeks or months. The strawberry marks then gradually fade and shrink, and, in almost all instances, are gone by age five or six.

Two uncommon but permanent birthmarks are port wine marks and pigmented moles. Both may be tiny or extensive and may be present anywhere on the skin. They grow in proportion to the growth of the child's body. Port wine marks are smooth, flat, and purplish. Pigmented moles are brown to black, often slightly raised, and may have dark hairs.

Diagnosis

Each type of birthmark is recognized by its typical appearance and behavior. Mongolian spots are not always immediately distinguishable from bruises until it becomes apparent that they are not fading.

Home Treatment

Strawberry marks are composed of countless, closely packed capillaries and may need to be protected from scratching or rubbing which can result in bleeding. If bleeding occurs it can be controlled by pressing lightly with gauze directly on the bleeding point. Port wine marks can be hidden by Covermark cosmetic or similar products when the child is older.

Precautions

● Strawberry marks occasionally become infected if the overlying skin is broken. Any discharge, odor, or redness of the surrounding skin should be reported to your doctor.
● Strawberry marks rarely require treatment; in almost all instances better results are obtained by allowing them to disappear spontaneously. In rare situations they may cause anemia or generalized spontaneous bleeding that requires correction.

Doctor's Treatment

Pigmented moles may require surgical removal. Strawberry marks rarely require surgical removal, irradiation, or oral steroids. Port wine marks cannot be treated satisfactorily at present, but laser treatment is being experimented with and appears promising.

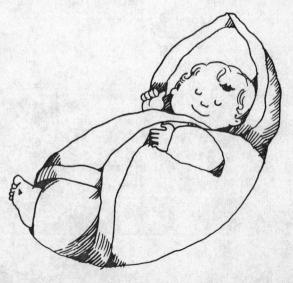

Birthmarks are as common as kisses; most marks fade in time.

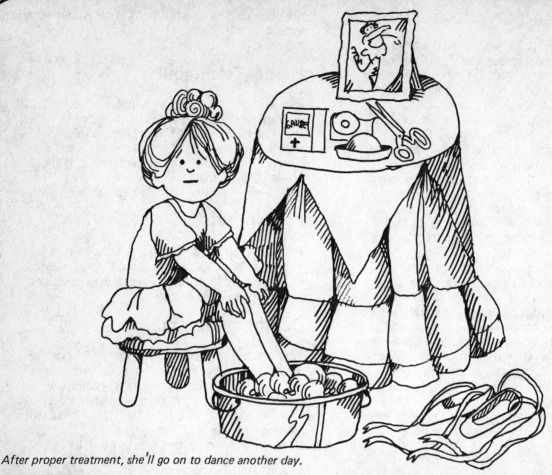

After proper treatment, she'll go on to dance another day.

Description

Blisters are an accumulation of clear or almost clear fluid between layers of the skin. They may be caused by: heat burns; chemical burns; rubbing (friction); infection by bacteria; viruses; hand, foot, and mouth disease; funguses; allergy to insect bites; or allergy to certain plants. Blisters range from the size of a pinhead to several inches.

Diagnosis

The cause of blisters is determined by taking a history and noting location and appearance. When blisters appear on the palms or heels they are usually due to friction (most blisters of the feet are caused by ill-fitting shoes and by not wearing socks); on the soles and toes they may be caused by a fungus; on cuticles of fingers or backs of fingers blisters almost always represent infection.

Home Treatment

Do not break open blisters caused by friction or burns. Protect them with gauze and bandages.

If accidentally opened, trim away the major portion of loose skin, cleanse with soap and water, and bandage. If the blister becomes infected (redness and increasing tenderness are signs of infection) it should be opened and soaked in an Epsom salt or Burrough's solution (available over-the-counter).

Precautions

● Red streaks spreading from a blister indicate spreading infection. ● Soaking unbroken blisters in too weak a solution causes marked enlargement of the blisters (suggested Epsom salts solution is at least four ounces salts to a quart of water).

Doctor's Treatment

Your doctor will confirm your diagnosis and evaluate the presence and severity of infection. Infected blisters are opened and the fluid cultured for type. Soaks or oral antibiotics may be prescribed individually or in combination.

Related Topics: Athlete's Foot; Blood Poisoning; Chicken Pox; Hand, Foot, & Mouth Disease; Herpes Simplex; Impetigo; Poison Ivy.

BLOOD POISONING

Description

Blood poisoning is the spread of a bacterial infection which has invaded the blood stream (septicemia) or of a viral infection (viremia). It is more apt to occur during early infancy when resistance is low. Beyond infancy, blood poisoning results in high fever, chills, and prostration.

In popular usage, blood poisoning refers to the red streaks that may develop from an infected wound or blister and quickly (within hours) extend in the direction of the heart. These red streaks, which resemble broad, wobbly, red-pencil marks, are signs of the infection traveling along the lymph vessels of the affected part of the body. If ignored, the spreading germs can—within hours or days—reach the bloodstream via the lymphatics.

In their trip along the lymph channels the germs encounter lymph nodes. The nodes swell and become tender and sometimes red as their cells engage and kill the germs. If the lymph nodes succeed in warding off the poisonous germs the infection is halted. No fever, or one below 100°F, indicates that the germs have not reached the bloodstream; a high, spiking fever (over 101°F) generally means they have.

Diagnosis

The pink or red, slightly wavy lines just under the skin, one inch to several feet in length, are unmistakable in a good light. The lymph nodes toward which these red streaks lead are often enlarged and tender.

Home Treatment

Elevate the affected part. Apply warm soaks of Epsom salts (one-half cup in a quart of water) to the entire area. If there is an unopened infected blister at the source, open it with a sterile needle to drain and include it in the soaks. Give aspirin or acetaminophen for pain and fever, following the dosage on the label.

Precautions

● Contact your doctor. Blood poisoning is best treated with antibiotics. ● If your child has a high fever or is prostrate **contact a medical facility promptly.**

Doctor's Treatment

Your doctor will give your child antibiotics by mouth or intravenously. The doctor may incise and drain the point of infection. Culture of the blood or from the site of the original infection may be necessary. Laboratory tests including a blood count and urinalysis may be required. Hospitalization may be necessary if the blood poisoning is severe.

Related Topic: Lymph Nodes—Infection Fighters

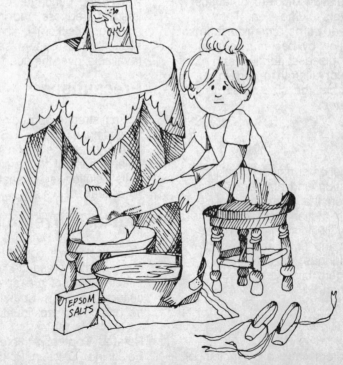

Watch for red, wavy lines aiming for the lymph nodes.

Description

Boils are localized infections that occur beneath the skin. With rare exception, they are caused by a bacterium called hemolytic staphylococcus aureus—"staph" for short. They are characterized by redness, pain, and the formation of pus in the center, which tends to "point" (come to a head) and drain through the skin. Pus is a mixture of live and dead white blood cells, liquified dead tissue, and live and dead staph germs. Pus is therefore infectious and can spread boils to other areas and to other persons.

A small superficial boil is a *pimple* or *pustule*. (An acne pimple or "zit" is not a true boil.) A large boil with multiple heads is a *carbuncle*. A boil on edges of the eyelids is a *stye*. When many boils are present at one time the condition is called *furunculosis*. Abcesses are collections of pus in parts other than the skin, as in muscles, brain, bone, and internal organs. They are equivalent to boils but often are caused by germs other than staph.

Staph germs are often harmlessly present in the nose and throat, and on the skin of well persons. They require a break in the skin to invade and cause infections.

Diagnosis

Diagnosis is determined by the presence of the above-mentioned symptoms.

Home Treatment

Boils respond to frequent or constant soaks with warm Epsom salts solutions (one-half cup per quart of water). When a boil comes to a head and drains, the drainage must be caught on a sterile bandage, and the surrounding skin should be cleansed frequently with soap and water to avoid secondary boils. Boils that have come to a head but not opened may be opened carefully with a sterilized needle, if your doctor agrees. Then the area should be soaked until all the pus, tenderness, and most of the redness is gone.

Precautions

● Be careful with boils on the face and forehead, including the nose and lips. The lymph and blood vessel drainage from these areas is partly internal. See your doctor.
● Never squeeze a boil. Squeezing disrupts the localizing wall formed by the body and may result in rapid spread of infection. ● Treat all minor wounds and insect bites properly to minimize the likelihood of boil formation.

Doctor's Treatment

Your doctor may incise and drain the boil, culture pus, and order sensitivity studies on the staph recovered to identify the antibiotic which will effectively fight the infection. Oral antibiotics will often be given. Many staph infections have become resistant to penicillin. Alternative antibiotics include erythromycin, oxacillin, cloxacillin, methicillin, and cephalosporin.

For chronic recurrent attacks of boils your doctor may recommend nose and throat cultures of the patient and the entire family to identify carriers. Intranasal antibiotic ointments and antiseptic baths may be prescribed. Your doctor may suggest immunization against staph by regular injections of dead staph vaccine for extended periods (months or years).

Related Topics: Acne, Cuts, Insect Bites, Puncture Wounds, Scrapes, Styes

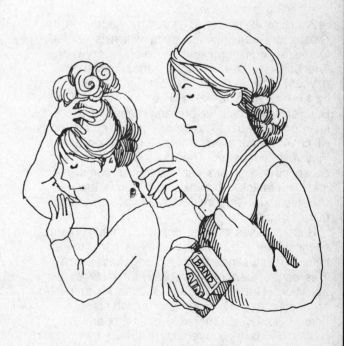

Boils respond well to Epsom salts soaks.

BOTULISM

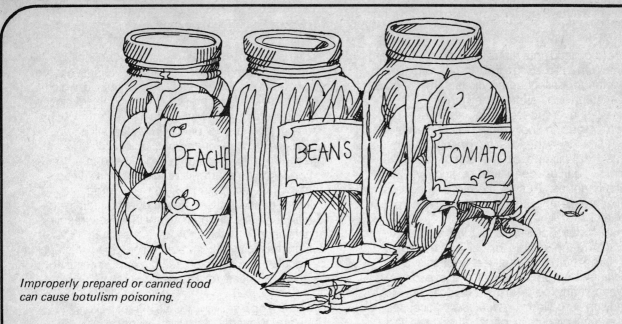

Improperly prepared or canned food can cause botulism poisoning.

Description

With improvements in commercial food preparation and the decline in home canning in the early to mid-20th century, botulism had become a rare illness in the United States. With the increased interest in "natural" foods (those without preservatives), botulism is threatening a comeback.

Botulism is caused by the toxin produced by Clostridium botulinum, a germ which is related to the tetanus germ and prevalent everywhere. The botulism germ grows in anaerobic (no oxygen) environments. Its toxin can be destroyed by an exposure to 180°F heat for 10 minutes. Botulism poisoning is primarily caused by improperly prepared, canned, or preserved foods which have not been adequately heated before they've been eaten. The most likely foods to cause poisoning are seafood, mushrooms, meat, and vegetables. The toxin and germs are undetectable. Contaminated foods look and taste normal.

Recent cases of fatal botulism among infants suggest that the germ of botulism can grow in immature intestines to form dangerous toxin. This cannot happen in adults who must swallow the toxin. The only natural food so far identified as a source of C. botulinum for infants is honey. However, other raw or improperly cooked foods may eventually surface as potential sources. Furthermore, indications that the Food and Drug Administration may outlaw nitrites as meat preservatives may make meats such as frankfurters and salami potential sources of botulism.

Symptoms of botulism are: nausea; vomiting; diarrhea; abdominal pain followed in 12 to 48 hours by double vision; dilated pupils; difficulty speaking, swallowing, and breathing. Fever is absent and no loss of awareness or alertness occurs. **Death may result.**

Diagnosis

Suspect botulism if your infant develops symptoms within a week of eating raw or home-prepared foods. Suspect the disease if more than one member of your family develops similar symptoms after eating the same prepared food. If symptoms of gastrointestinal upset are followed by paralysis that starts at eyes and descends, botulism may be the cause. Home diagnosis, however, is totally unreliable. Consult your doctor.

Home Treatment

None.

Precautions

● Do not give babies unwashed, unpeeled and raw or improperly cooked foods. ● Do not use foods in damaged, store-bought cans. ● When canning or preserving foods at home, follow preparation directions carefully.

Doctor's Treatment

Diagnosis is established by cultures of the food eaten, stomach contents, and stools and by identification of toxin in the patient's blood. Treatment includes injection of the antitoxin, stomach washing, laxatives and enemas, possibly antibiotics, and hospitalization. Preventative immunization is available for persons at high risk.

BOWLEGS AND KNOCK~KNEES

Description

Theoretically, when a child stands at attention his ankle bones should touch each other and his knee bones should touch each other. With an infant on his stomach or back, the legs can be pulled straight with the toes and knees pointed straight ahead to determine the relationship of the knee and ankle bones. If the ankles touch but the knees do not, the child can be said to be bowlegged. If the knees touch but the ankles do not, he is knock-kneed.

However, by these criteria all infants, children, and adults are bowlegged or knock-kneed to some degree. Most infants appear bowlegged until they walk, and when they start to walk they do so "cowboy" style. This condition usually corrects itself by age two. Most preschoolers stand knock-kneed, especially if they are plump. This condition corrects itself.

True bowlegs and knock-knees are either due to rickets (vitamin D deficiency) or are developmental (genetic). Common 50 and more years ago, rickets is now rare in the United States. An unusual form of bowlegs, often one-sided and probably developmental, is Blount's disease, in which the near end of the tibia (shin bone) becomes deformed.

Diagnosis

Diagnosis is made by having the child stand with his legs straight and his toes pointed forward and measuring any distance between the knees or ankles. The average breadth is only a finger's width or two, but it is such an individual thing that no criteria for whether or not the legs are abnormal is helpful.

Home Treatment

In most cases, no treatment is needed. To prevent rickets, all children should receive about 400 international units of vitamin D daily. This amount is present in many commercial formulas, and in most commercial milk. Some vitamin D is present in breast milk.

Precautions

● If you think your infant or child is bowlegged or knock-kneed, watch to see if, after several months, the condition worsens. If it does, consult your doctor. ● Do not use orthopedic shoes without your doctor's prescription.

Doctor's Treatment

In most instances, your doctor will evaluate your child and then prescribe no treatment—except to wait and watch. X rays of the knees may be required as well as a test for rickets or refractory rickets (blood tests). Use of orthopedic shoes or night splints is rarely necessary. In Blount's disease, braces or corrective operations on bones may be required.

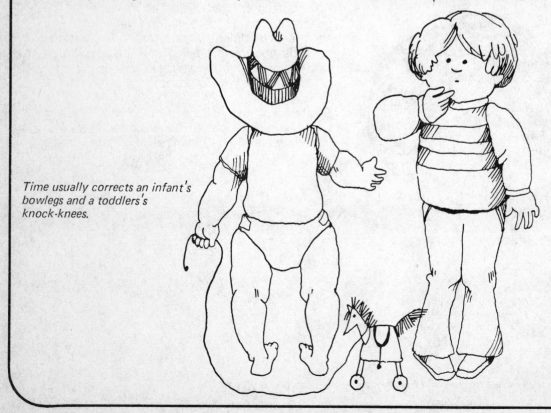

Time usually corrects an infant's bowlegs and a toddlers's knock-knees.

BREATHING DIFFICULTY

Description

There are many illnesses that cause difficulty in breathing including asthma, bronchiolitis, diphtheria, colds, croup, hay fever, and pneumonia. In addition there is a condition that causes the sensation of difficult breathing that is not a physical illness at all. It is called *air hunger* or the *hyperventilation syndrome*, and it is common in older children, adolescents, and young adults. The patient complains, often bitterly or fearfully, of being unable to "get enough air" while at the same time taking deep breaths in and out with no visible difficulty. The rate of breathing may be rapid or normal. There is no abnormal sound to the breathing as in croup, bronchitis, or asthma. Temperature and color are both normal, and there is no cough. In fact, the deep breathing can be recognized as sighing, one sigh right after another, lasting for minutes or hours. The cause is essentially the same as that of sighing; nervous tension, fear, anxiety, or depression.

If the hyperventilation continues long enough, the patient will experience tingling and numbness in the hands and feet, followed by spasms of the muscles that control the hands, fingers, ankles, and toes. This is caused by alkalosis due to the blowing off of too much CO_2. If hyperventilation continues long enough, convulsions and unconsciousness can occur.

Unconsciousness temporarily cures the condition, and the patient recovers.

Diagnosis

Close observation will determine that your child is having no trouble getting copious breaths of air in and out. Hyperventilation syndrome is never accompanied by cough or fever. Susceptible children may have recurrent attacks.

Home Treatment

Your reassurance and calmness are essential. Have your child breathe into a large paper bag held loosely over his mouth and nose. This will allow him to rebreathe the exhaled carbon dioxide. Mild tranquilizers are permissible with your doctor's approval. Look for such causes as intolerable pressures or anxieties in the child's environment at home, at school, and among peer relationships.

Precautions

● Hyperventilation syndrome can develop as a result of rapid, prolonged, forced, deep breathing which has become a party stunt in some circles. Convulsions and injuries from falls can result. Encourage other kinds of games.

Doctor's Treatment

Acute attack will be treated as in home treatment. Tranquilizers may be used for short-term treatment. Fundamental treatment depends upon investigating and analyzing your child's environment. Psychiatric counseling may be advised for severe cases.

Related Topics: Asthma, Bronchiolitis, Choking, Common Cold, Croup, Funnel Chest, Hay Fever, Pneumonia, Shortness of Breath

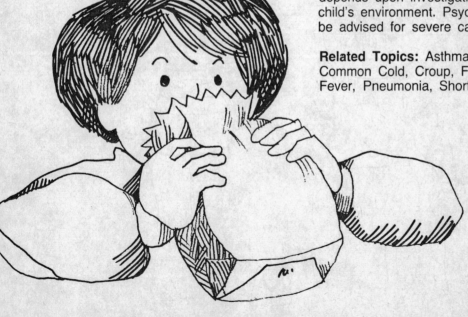

Breathing into a paper bag allows a child to inhale the exhaled carbon dioxide.

Description

There is a question whether this is a different disease than bronchitis, or merely bronchitis altered by the young age and other considerations peculiar to the child. Bronchiolitis occurs during the first two years of life, with peak incidence at about six months of age. It is almost always caused by a respiratory virus, especially the syncytial virus, but also by parainfluenza viruses, mycoplasma, and adenoviruses.

Early symptoms are similar to those of bronchitis and often appear after exposure to an older child or adult with a cold. They are nasal congestion, fever of 102°F, loss of appetite, and a mild cough. These symptoms then progress to: frequent, severe coughing; rapid and difficult breathing; wheezing; irritability; cyanosis (a bluish discoloration especially of the skin); flaring of the nostrils, and retractions of the spaces between the ribs and of the abdomen immediately beneath the ribs because of the effort of breathing. The illness may last for weeks. As with bronchitis, infants subject to bronchiolitis may develop asthma or other allergies in later years.

Diagnosis

Diagnosis is determined by observation of the above symptoms.

Home Treatment

Diagnosis and treatment should be handled by your doctor. See your doctor if your infant has a frequent cough of any duration or if your child has difficulty in breathing other than that caused by nasal obstruction or hyperventilation syndrome. Home treatment, if recommended by your doctor, is similar to that of bronchitis.

Precautions

• Bronchiolitis is a dangerous illness.
• Cough medicines may be dangerous to a child who is already having difficulty breathing.
• An infant with rapid breathing can become dehydrated from loss of vapor in the breath. He requires extra fluids by mouth.

Doctor's Treatment

In some areas bronchiolitis is the most common reason for hospitalizing infants. An infant with bronchiolitis may require oxygen therapy, high humidity, or intravenous fluids; a chest X ray, nose and throat cultures, and a blood count may be ordered. The use of antibiotics and steroids is dubious. One injection of epinephrine may be given to rule out allergy.

Related Topics: Asthma, Bronchitis, Common Cold, Frequent Illnesses, Viruses

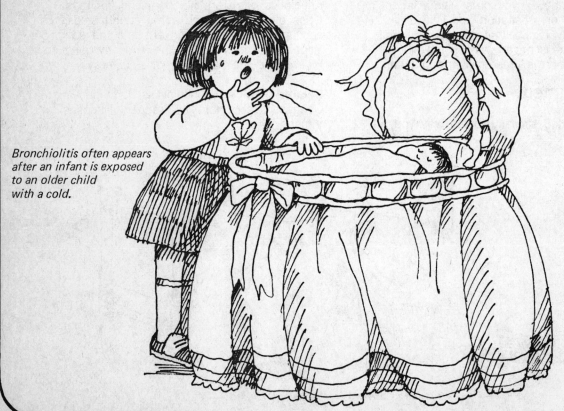

Bronchiolitis often appears after an infant is exposed to an older child with a cold.

BRONCHITIS

Description

Bronchitis may be thought of as a cold that spreads to the windpipe (trachea) and bronchial tubes. It may start with signs of a common upper respiratory cold with nasal congestion and discharge, sneezing, watery eyes, and scratchy throat. Bronchitis may also develop without any preceding cold symptoms.

The condition is characterized by a dry, hacking cough; a low-grade (100°F, oral; 101°F, rectal) or no fever; and tightness and pain in the front, center of the chest. Loss of appetite and a general feeling of malaise are common. After a few days the cough loosens. Occasionally, a rattling sound can be heard in the chest when the child takes a breath, but there is never any real difficulty in breathing. The entire course of the condition may last more than a week.

Most cases are caused by one of many viruses. These viruses do not respond to antibiotics. Bronchitis is contagious and is passed on in the same manner as a cold. If the disease recurs frequently it may indicate that the child has an underlying allergy. (Sometimes children with asthma are unusually susceptible to recurrent attacks of bronchitis.)

Diagnosis

Diagnosis is determined by the presence or absence of the above symptoms. There is rarely high fever or prostration and little or no breathing difficulty except that caused by nasal obstruction. There is never pain on the side of the chest. No blood is present in the sputum.

Home Treatment

Bronchitis is treated similarly to the way you would treat a common cold. Limited activity is recommended during the fever stage and the worst of the cough. Give aspirin or acetaminophen for fever and malaise. Phenylephrine or oxymetazoline nose drops may be used. A humidifier or vaporizer aids breathing. Cough medicine at bedtime or for an exhausting cough can be helpful. Encourage your child to drink liquids to avoid dehydration.

Precautions

● See your doctor if any unusual symptoms occur such as pain on the side of the chest or blood in the sputum. ● See your doctor if bronchitis recurs more than once a year. ● See your doctor if the condition worsens instead of improving after three to four days. ● Avoid the use of oral decongestants which may tighten the chest and aggravate a dry cough.

Doctor's Treatment

Your child's physical examination should include a careful examination of his chest. Throat or sputum cultures, a chest X ray, and blood count may be taken. If bronchitis is recurrent your doctor will investigate allergy possibilities, the chance of a foreign body being in the bronchial tubes, or the presence of diminished immune mechanisms. The use of antibiotics and some types of cough medicines is debatable. Antibiotics often are not beneficial for most types of bronchitis and some cough medicines can aggravate more than alleviate the condition. Your doctor may give epinephrine by injection to evaluate the possibility of an allergy.

Related Topics: Bronchiolitis, Common Cold, Coughs, Cystic Fibrosis, Frequent Illnesses, Viruses

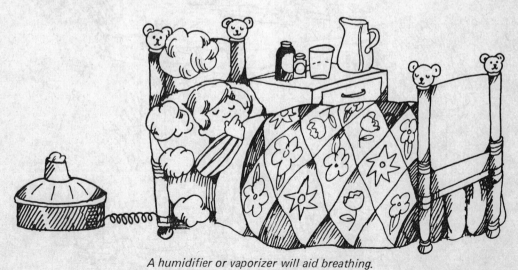

A humidifier or vaporizer will aid breathing.

BRUISES

Description

Bruises consist of blood that has escaped from capillaries or larger blood vessels and is visible through the skin. They vary from pinhead-size to several inches in diameter, and usually are black and blue in color; if they are near the skin's surface they appear maroon or purple. Bruises of the whites of the eyeballs are always blood-red. As blood is reabsorbed, bruises often become yellow or green. If the escape of blood has been deep in the tissues—as with torn ligaments or broken bones—it may take days to reach the skin's surface as a visible bruise. Escaped blood often travels to other parts of the body. For example, a bruise of the forehead may travel to form black eyes.

Most bruises are caused by physical trauma. Most normally active children always seem to have one or more bruises. Fair-complected children bruise more easily than dark-complected ones. Particularly vulnerable are the shins, knees, arms, and thighs. Bruises take days or weeks to disappear depending upon their size.

Bruises that appear spontaneously are cause for concern. These often appear in areas and in numbers that defy the likelihood that the cause has gone unnoticed. Spontaneous bruises result from abnormally fragile capillaries (e.g., scurvy or vitamin C deficiency), capillaries injured by infections or by allergic reactions, or from a deficiency of the clotting mechanisms of the blood.

There is one type of bruise known as a *petechia*. Petechiae are pinhead to one-eighth inch in size, dark red or maroon in color, and are often present by the hundreds. Petechiae may appear from the neck up from forceful vomiting or coughing or in localized area when caused by a blow.

Diagnosis

A bruise of any size does not blanch when pressed upon, as do all other red or purple marks or rashes of the skin.

Home Treatment

Cold applications soon after the injury has occurred decrease bleeding and minimize bruising. *Warm* applications 24 or more hours afterward hasten reabsorption of the bruise.

Precautions

● Spontaneous bruising should always be evaluated by a doctor. ● Petechiae scattered over the body can indicate an **urgent situation.** If fever or prostration is present, a true emergency exists. Don't waste any time; see your doctor at once.

Doctor's Treatment

For traumatic bruises, a doctor's treatment is the same as the home treatment. Your doctor may prescribe an oral enzyme—streptokinase-streptodornase—which can speed absorption of some bruises. For spontaneous bruises, including generalized petechiae, your doctor will give a complete physical examination including: blood count; platelet count; blood coagulation studies; nose, throat, and blood cultures; spinal tap; and bone marrow studies. The patient may be hospitalized for administration of intravenous fluids and oral steroids and antibiotic therapy.

Related Topics: Leukemia, Meningitis

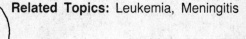
Active children always seem to have bruises.

BURNS

Description

Burns are injuries of the skin caused by excessive heat (thermal burns), acids and alkalis, or electricity. Depth, extent, and location of the burn are important. Superficial burns (*first-degree*) cause reddening of the skin and pain; they may blister after one to two days. (Sunburn is a good example of a first-degree burn.) *Second-degree* burns redden and blister immediately. *Third-degree* burns are deepest and involve the death of a full depth of skin. The skin blisters or appears scorched (blackened) or dead white. The actual depth of a burn, except mild first-degree and severe third-degree conditions, cannot be reliably determined until healing starts.

Skin is a vital organ. If more than ten percent of the skin area has suffered second- or third-degree burns a serious emergency exists. If an area larger than twice the size of a child's palm receives a second-degree burn or any size area suffers a third-degree burn consult your doctor. Burns of the fingers, joints, and face are threatening because of danger of scarring and deformity.

Diagnosis

Redness, blistering, or scorching of the skin constitutes a burn. The problem is in deciding the degree and extent of the burn. Burns with no blistering or charring can be assumed to be first-degree.

Home Treatment

Immediately apply cold water compresses to the burn. If the burn is a first-degree type, continue applications until the pain abates or up to one-half hour. If the burn is serious cover it with a clean, cold, wet cloth; keep your child warm; and see your doctor at once. Do not apply ointments or other treatments to burns that will need a doctor's care.

Although some hospital burn centers treat burns by the open (uncovered) method under sterilized conditions, home treatment of a first-degree burn (other than sunburn which may be treated with OTC preparations) consists of applying a nonadherent dressing that will exclude air and germs until the burn has healed. (Once air is excluded from the burn, there should be no further pain.) Apply petroleum jelly or a cream containing silver sulfadiazine liberally to the burn and cover the area with several thicknesses of sterile gauze. Change the dressing every 24 to 48 hours until the burn completely heals.

Precautions

• Burns are the second leading cause of accidental death among children under age four and the third leading cause among older children. **Prevention is paramount.** • Water over 115°F can scald. Homes with children should have aquastats turned low. (The temperature of boiling water is 212°F.) • Keep matches and cigarette lighters out of your child's reach as they should be considered deadly poisons. • Do not keep gasoline or other inflammables in the home. Keep under lock and key outside. • Avoid inflammable garments. • Keep child-proof plugs in electrical outlets. • Serious electrical burns are common as a result of young children chewing live electrical wires and extension cords. • Second- and third-degree burns require up-to-date tetanus boosters.

Doctor's Treatment

Your doctor will usually hospitalize your child for third-degree burns, second-degree burns that cover more than ten percent of the skin, and for second-degree burns of the face, fingers, or joints. Burns covering more than 30 percent of the body usually require treatment at specialized burn centers.

Hospital treatment involves proper dressings, close attention to the need for intravenous fluids, attention to kidney and stomach complications, and sometimes antibiotics and plastic surgery.

Related Topic: Sunburn

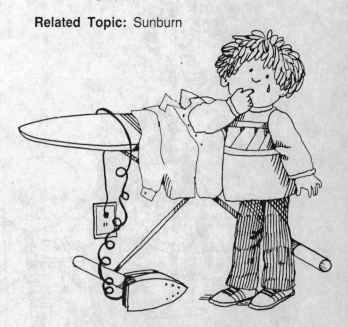

Prevent burns wherever possible. They're a threat to children of all ages.

CAT SCRATCH FEVER

Description

Cat scratch fever is caused by a germ—probably a virus—contracted by a superficial scratch or bite from a kitten or young cat. The cat is not ill. The puncture wound or scratch does not heal in the time expected and one to two weeks later is still red, sometimes with a small amount of pus. One to six weeks after the incident, the lymph nodes of the area become swollen, tender, red, and there is a low-grade fever (100°F, oral; 101°F, rectal). Eventually the lymph glands may break down and discharge pus through the skin.

Diagnosis

Diagnosis is made by history, presence of a minor wound that hasn't healed, and the development of large, tender lymph nodes. If you don't know that your child has been scratched by a cat this condition may be confused with a wound infected with staph or tuberculosis germs.

Home Treatment

Wash all cat scratches and bites with soap and water as soon as possible and apply an antiseptic. If the wound becomes infected see your doctor.

Precautions

● Unsupervised play between cats and young children is dangerous to both the child and the cat. ● Tormenting of cats by older children can readily result in a scratch and requires investigation of the child's emotional state.

Doctor's Treatment

Your doctor will rule out other illnesses by blood tests and cultures. Treatment with broad-spectrum antibiotics is occasionally beneficial. Cat scratch fever may require surgical incision and drainage or the complete removal of an involved lymph gland.

Related Topic: Lymph Nodes—Infection Fighters

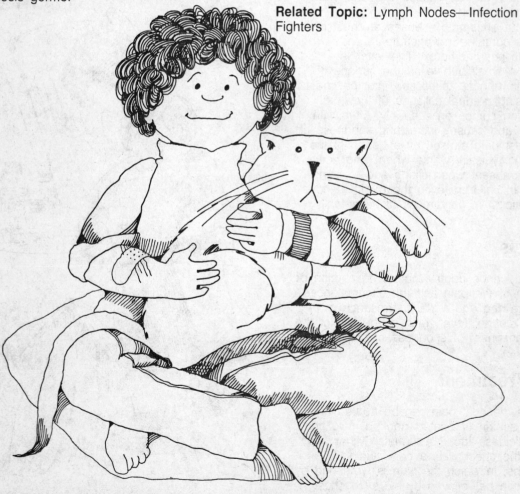

Wash a cat scratch right away; apply an antiseptic.

CHEST PAIN

Description

Chest pain is common during childhood. Contrary to that which occurs in adults, it is rarely a symptom of serious disease. A frequent form is the so-called stitch in the side—a stabbing pain in the lower anterior (front) chest, more often on the left side than the right. This pain occurs with exercise and will cease after a minute or two of rest. Various explanations include gas pains in the large intestine, contraction of the spleen, and spasm of the diaphragm. In any event, it is harmless.

Pain in the area of the sternum (breastbone) is common with bronchitis and with a head cold combined with a cough. Also common is pain at the rib margins from a sore diaphragm caused by a frequent, hard cough. One-sided chest pain accompanies pleurodynia, and shingles.

Injuries, including muscle strains, bruises, and fractured ribs cause pain aggravated by deep breathing and movements of the chest. All of the above are relatively nonserious and often can be home treated.

Serious but uncommon causes of chest pain are pleurisy complicating pneumonia and spontaneous pneumothorax. The latter is a bursting of a small bubble on the surface of the lung, allowing air to escape into the chest cavity, causing gradual collapse of the lung. This condition comes on suddenly, often with sharp pain, and causes increasing shortness of breath. Chest pain caused by a hernia of the diaphragm is typically worse when lying down, and less or absent when sitting and standing. Heart pain in children, even those with serious heart conditions, is so rare as to be virtually unknown.

Diagnosis

Diagnosis depends upon accurate description of the location of the pain and the circumstances that provoke and aggravate it. Presence or absence of cough, fever, rash at the site of the pain, and an onset of shortness of breath are all clues.

Home Treatment

Most cases of chest pain can be treated at home with aspirin or acetaminophen, mild heat, cough medicines, and reassurance. Minor injuries of the chest wall, even including fractured ribs, in which the pain is worsened by breathing, can be relieved by a Velcro chest bandage, available at pharmacies and hospital supply stores.

Precautions

● Chest pain accompanied by shortness of breath, high fever, a cough producing blood flecks, or prostration requires **prompt medical attention.** ● Persistent pain beneath either armpit aggravated by breathing also should be evaluated by your doctor.

Doctor's Treatment

Your doctor may require X rays and blood tests. Pneumothorax is treated by hospitalization, close observation, and possibly a puncture of the chest wall to remove trapped air.

Related Topics: Bronchitis, Pneumonia, Shingles, Viruses

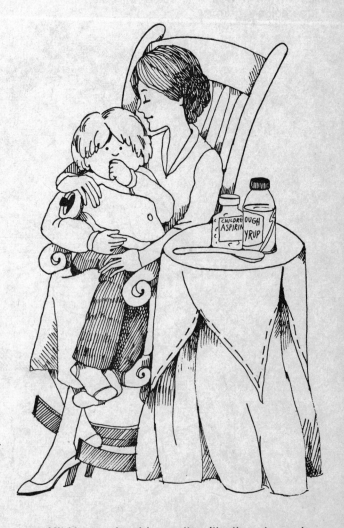

Mild heat and aspirin usually will relieve chest pain.

CHICKEN POX

Description

Chicken pox is caused by a specific virus which is highly contagious. The disease is contracted through the air from a person in the same room. There are no carriers. No one is naturally immune, not even newborn babies, but one attack gives lifelong immunity unless the attack is extremely mild. The incubation period is 14 to 16 days. There is no immunization available.

Chicken pox may start with the symptoms of a mild cold, but usually a rash is the first sign. The rash worsens for three to four days, then heals in three to four days. The child is contagious from 24 hours before the rash appears until all blisters of the rash have dried. Fever can be low or as high as 105°F; fever is the worst on the third or fourth day after rash appears.

Diagnosis

Diagnosis is made from the typical appearance of the rash. At first, each new spot resembles an insect bite, but within hours develops a small, clear blister in the center which may be hard to see without good light. Most blisters break and are replaced by a brown scab. The rash is distributed randomly all over the skin including the scalp, and on the mucous membranes of the mouth, genitalia, anus, and eyelids. It becomes quite itchy. It never appears in bunches or groups. New lesions continue to appear hour by hour for three to four days. No other rash has all these characteristics.

Home Treatment

Bed rest is not required, but your child should be isolated from others. Cut his fingernails to minimize the scratching. To reduce the itching give antihistamines or hydroxyzines by mouth, bathe your child in a tepid water-with-corn-starch bath, and apply calamine lotion to the skin with a soft brush. Anesthetic ointment may be applied to sore poxes around the anus and genitalia. Give aspirin or acetaminophen for fever or pain.

Precautions

● Chicken pox is dangerous to young babies, to patients on steroids or other immunosuppressant drugs, and to those with immune mechanism deficiencies. Report any known exposures or the onset of chicken pox in such children to your doctor. ● Even though a sibling may already have been exposed, prevent further exposure because severity of the illness increases with the length of exposure. ● Encephalitis is a rare complication; if high fever, prostration, headache, vomiting and convulsions occur, see your doctor. ● The pox may become infected, showing an increasing redness, soreness, and formation of pus. The lymph glands of the neck, armpits, groin, and back of the skull swell with chicken pox, but if they become red and tender they may be secondarily infected; report this to your doctor. ● DO NOT apply calamine with phenol. ● When your child is bathed, pat him dry without breaking the blisters or disturbing the scabs to avoid scarring. ● If spontaneous bruising or ruptured blood vessels under the skin appear, see your doctor.

Doctor's Treatment

Your doctor will usually culture an infected pox and will treat your child with oral antibiotics for five to ten days. (Antibiotics do not influence the *course* of the chicken pox, however.) If your child is at high risk (see above) and is exposed to chicken pox, your doctor will probably give him a zoster immune globulin or a gamma globulin shot. If there are signs of encephalitis, your child will probably be hospitalized for tests and treatment. Spontaneous bleeding under the skin may be treated with oral medications or your doctor may request hospitalization.

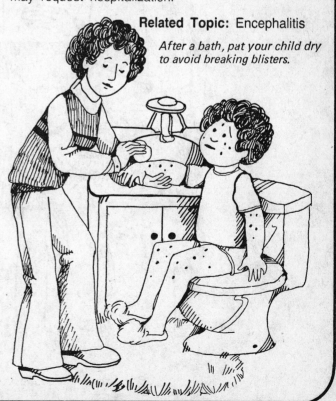

Related Topic: Encephalitis

After a bath, pat your child dry to avoid breaking blisters.

CHOKING

Description

Choking is one of the few true emergencies of childhood in which minutes may determine life or death. There are only two causes: croup, especially bacterial, and foreign substances obstructing the airway.

Choking must be distinguished from gagging which is much more common but not nearly as serious. Gagging is caused by a tickling or irritation of the throat or as a prelude to vomiting. There is only momentary interference with breathing, speaking, or crying. Choking is caused by the inability to take a breath and is readily identified by the sustained frantic efforts to breathe and by the inability of the child to cry out or to speak.

Breath-holding and a temporary stoppage of breathing during a convulsion may resemble choking; in breath-holding there is no effort made to breathe. At the onset of a convulsion the child often cries out; there is no effort to breathe at first, and then breathing, though erratic, returns.

If choking continues the child quickly becomes blue, convulsive, limp, and unconscious. **If the obstruction is complete you have between five and ten minutes to reestablish an airway before death occurs.**

The objects that choke children are usually of a shape and size to plug the opening into the larynx like a cork. Notorious items are peanuts, tablets, glass eyes of toy animals, hard or hard-coated candies, beads, popcorn, and tiny toys or small parts from toys. Solid particles of food from the stomach may choke a child who breathes in during vomiting. A baby who vomits is safest from choking if he is lying on his stomach. A child may choke temporarily on liquids that "go down the wrong tube," but spontaneous coughing and deep breaths quickly relieve the problem.

Diagnosis

The diagnosis depends on identifying the situation correctly according to the above description. There is frantic, unsuccessful effort to breathe. The child is silent.

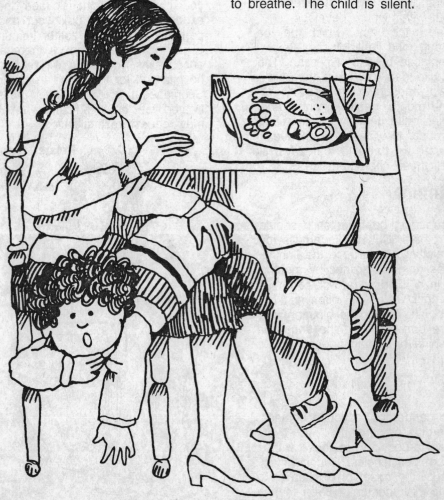

Four sharp blows on the back may clear the obstruction.

CHOKING

Home Treatment

Seconds count! Scream for help. A second adult on the scene should phone the police or paramedic squad for help. (Police are usually more quickly available in most communities than an ambulance, the fire department, or a doctor.)

First, give your child one minute to clear the obstruction by his or her own efforts. If this doesn't work place your child head down over a chair, table, or your lap and pound hard on his back four times. Broken ribs heal, death does not. A baby may be held upside down by the ankles, but **always** support head and neck before pounding to avoid fracturing the neck.

If this is unsuccessful try the maneuver shown in the adjacent art. While standing to the child's back, press or squeeze vigorously and sharply on lower rib margins below the breastbone. You are trying to compress the upper abdomen and lower chest and to force the diaphragm up swiftly so that air in the lungs will pop the object causing the obstruction from the airway. Only if these safer measures fail should you consider reaching into the child's throat with a hooked finger or tweezers in an effort to remove or dislodge the foreign body: there's a good chance of driving the object more tightly into the windpipe in your desperation to remove it. If your child is not breathing after the object is removed, give mouth-to-mouth resuscitation until trained help arrives.

Precautions

- See precautions for choking due to croup.
- Never give mouth-to-mouth resuscitation until the obstructing object is removed; to do so may force the object further down the throat.
- Prevention of choking by foresight is most important: Examine all toys for loose eyes or other parts. Keep tablets under lock and key.
- Peanuts, popcorn, or hard candies should not be given to toddlers. (Clean up after adult parties before children can wande unattended into a room.) • Plastic bags must be kept out of reach of small children.

Doctor's Treatment

When the obstruction is complete, the child seldom reaches a doctor in time. The obstruction may be incomplete even though you may not think so. Your doctor will operate, on the spot, to open the windpipe through the neck (tracheostomy). Then oxygen, artificial respiration, intravenous fluids, and blood tests will be administered.

Related Topic: Croup

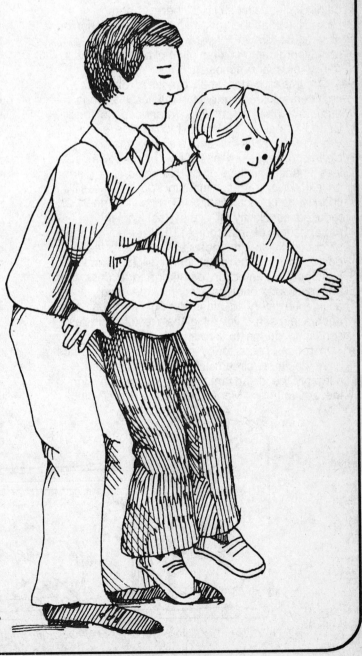

Squeezing sharply and vigorously below the breastbone may force the object out of the air passage.

CIRCUMCISION

Description

Circumcision is the removal of the foreskin of the penis. Most boy babies have a cuff of skin (foreskin) that covers the end of the penis (the glans). The natural opening in this cuff is generally large enough to allow urine through, but in a condition called *phimosis* it is not large enough to allow the foreskin to be pulled back to uncover the glans. Rarely is there no opening at all. When the opening in this cuff is too small to allow retraction, the foreskin can be stretched to sufficient size. It is desirable to expose the glans so that the normal, waxy material that forms under the foreskin (smegma) can be removed during bathing. If uncircumcised, there is some possibility that the retracted foreskin will not be able to be drawn forward again and may act as a tourniquet, cutting off the blood supply to the glans (paraphimosis).

Circumcision has been practiced on all continents for centuries for religious reasons and as a ritual to attaining manhood. In the United States it has been fashionable since World War II. Its advantages are: easier cleansing; lessened possibility of paraphimosis; less chance of developing cancer of the glans, an extremely rare malignancy; possibly less chance of cervical cancer of sexual partner; and reduced sensitivity of glans (resulting in prolongation of intercourse). The disadvantages of circumcision are: hospital expenses; fee of doctor or religious practitioner; slight chance of postoperative infection or hemorrhage (less than one percent); brief pain of the operation; rare, accidental injury to glans during operation; and decreased sensitivity of glans (resulting in less sensation during intercourse).

In recent years many professors of pediatrics have declared circumcision an unwarranted surgery, the disadvantages of which outweigh the advantages. Many experienced, practicing pediatricians feel that the advantages outweigh the disadvantages. The decision remains with the parents.

Diagnosis

Circumcision is *required* only in boys who are born with no opening in the foreskin, with an opening too small to allow passage of urine, or when paraphimosis has developed and must be immediately corrected.

Home Treatment

A circumcision wound should be covered, until healed (two to five days), with a nonadhering bandage and gauze covered with petroleum jelly. The area should not be submerged in bath water until the wound has healed.

Precautions

● Any bleeding of the circumcised penis in excess of a few drops should be reported to your doctor. ● Any evidence of infection (pus, spreading redness, the swelling of the shaft of the penis) should be evaluated by your doctor. ● Any residual cuff of skin left after circumcision should be pulled back to expose the base of the glans and this area should be cleansed during bathing. ● Boy babies born with malformations of the penis should not be circumcised because the foreskin may be necessary for future use in surgical correction of the malformation.

Doctor's Treatment

Your doctor (or religious leader) will perform the circumcision selecting from a wide variety of approved techniques. Ask for specific directions for care of the circumcision. In a rare instance of postoperative infection, the doctor will culture the wound and blood, and start antibiotics. (In some cultures female infants and women are also circumcised, removing the foreskin of the clitoris. This practice is rare in the United States.)

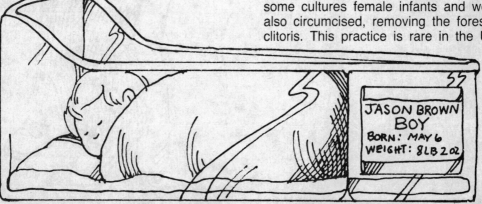

Debate about the advisability of circumcising infants persists; parents must make the decision.

Description

The word colic means any cramp-like, intermittent, abdominal pain. There are a variety of causes for all age groups. Infantile colic, or "three-month colic," is a specific problem that bothers ten to twenty percent of American babies. This form of colic starts during the first few weeks of life and lasts one to six months, (an average of three months). It takes the form of severe cramps of the digestive tract. An affected baby cries inconsolably for hours a day, particularly late afternoon and evening. He pulls his legs up, clenches his fists, screams, and turns red. He may nurse briefly but stops to return to crying. Rocking and cuddling interrupt the cries only briefly. In other respects the infant is normal; he gains weight well, has normal bowel movements, and doesn't spit up any more than most.

A variation of this classical form of colic is the infant past two weeks of age who wakes frequently (every two hours or so) cries fretfully, takes one to two ounces of formula or a few minutes at the mother's breast, falls into a fitful sleep, and wakens to repeat the sequence.

Diagnosis

Diagnosis depends upon investigating and ruling out other probable causes. Although it's virtually impossible to pinpoint the cause of crying in babies this young, if the symptoms are evident and the treatment for colic brings relief, the condition is colic.

Home Treatment

Check for obvious causes of discomfort other than colic: diarrhea or constipation; loose diaper pins; severe diaper rash; trapped arm or leg; whether baby is too hot or too cold; or signs of illness—fever, nasal discharge, cough, inflamed eyes, vomiting, hernia (lump in groin), or sores on the body. See whether your baby responds promptly to talking and cuddling and remains comfortable. (A baby in pain can be distracted but only temporarily.) If breast-feeding, check that your nipples are not bleeding. Swallowed blood causes cramps. Offer your baby a bottle even if he has been fed recently and even if breast-fed. If your baby drinks generously and falls asleep comfortably for several hours, he was hungry, not colicky. Keep the baby partially upright in an infant carrier between feedings to rule out regurgitation of food into the esophagus.

If colic still seems likely, temporary relief can be given using gentle heat on the abdomen or a pacifier. Also try inserting a glycerine suppository, soap stick, or lubricated thermometer to induce a bowel movement.

Precautions

● Make sure the formula is properly prepared. ● When bottle feeding your baby, be sure that the nipple is kept full to protect your baby from swallowing excessive air. ● Make sure the nipple holes are large enough so that he will be satisfied in a reasonable time (less than 20 to 25 minutes). ● Burp the baby carefully in different positions after each feeding.

Doctor's Treatment

Your doctor will check for signs of illness—sores in mouth and urinary tract problems, for example. (A urinalysis may be ordered.) Your doctor also may recommend a change in formula to investigate the possibility of formula intolerance and will temporarily stop any solids already started to rule out food intolerance. An anticolic medicine will be tried for one to three days. Stomach relaxants may be given at each feeding or only at feedings near the times that the attacks of colic usually occur. In proper dosage these medications will usually stop the discomfort of colic promptly (within one or two days). Generally, they will not stop pain from other causes, however, thus confirming the diagnosis of colic and treating it at the same time.

Related Topics: Constipation, Diarrhea in Infants, Fever, Hernia, Vomiting

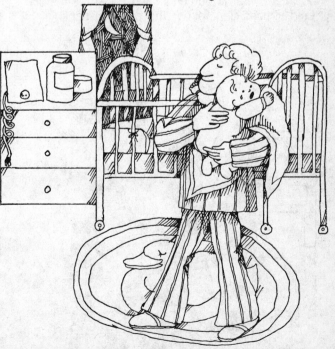

Cuddling provides only temporary relief from colic.

COMMON COLD

Description

A cold is a viral infection of the upper respiratory tract. It usually involves discomfort of the throat, nose, and paranasal sinuses, and sometimes the eyes (connected to the nose by the tear ducts), the ears (connected to the nose by the eustachian tubes), and the lymph nodes of the neck (connected by lymphatic channels). A cold is transmitted from person to person through the air, or via droplets on the hands and inanimate objects (toys, drinking glasses, handkerchiefs). The incubation period is two to seven days. People of all ages are susceptible, but younger children and infants are particularly at risk.

Symptoms of a cold are nasal congestion, sneezing, clear nasal discharge, scratchy-sore throat, and fever up to 103°F. (In general, the younger the child, the higher the fever.) Symptoms may also include reddened, watery eyes; dry cough; mild swelling and tenderness of cervical lymph nodes; stuffiness; and mild pain in the ears.

Many fruitless years had been spent attempting to develop a vaccine against the cold germ before it was discovered that the germ is actually many different viruses, and all respiratory viruses can cause common colds. An attack by any of the more than 185 viruses confers immunity against only that virus and none of the others and often only for a short time.

Many "cold viruses" can cause such complications as croup, laryngitis, bronchitis, bronchiolitis, viral pneumonia, and encephalitis. All cold viruses can render the child susceptible to secondary bacterial complications—ear infections, sinusitis, lymphadenitis, bacterial pneumonia. So no child's cold should be taken lightly.

Diagnosis

It is impossible to diagnose a common cold with certainty. Confirming viral cultures and antibody studies are possible, but the cost is prohibitive. The diagnosis is usually guessed from familiar symptoms, and absence of findings of other diseases, and by the fact that the ailment only lasts three to ten days and is gone.

Home Treatment

Give aspirin or acetaminophen for fever or pain. Use nose drops or oral decongestants and a nasal aspirator to relieve nasal stuffiness and discharge. Use cough medicines for easing a cough. Increase room humidity with a vaporizer or humidifier. Have your child drink a lot of liquids. Isolate him from others, particularly infant siblings and the elderly. Bed rest is not required, but do not allow strenuous physical activities while fever is present. Chest rubs and vitamin C treatments have not proven beneficial. Your child should eat only what he is able to.

Precautions

• The following symptoms are usually absent with a common cold: fever lasting more than two to three days; pus-like discharge from eyes, nose, ears; large, red, tender, neck glands; breathing difficulties; chest pain; severe headache; stiff neck; vomiting; shaking chills; and prostration. • Some viruses that cause commom colds are present in the body for one to two weeks so the child remains contagious for the entire course of the cold. • An infant is not protected against the common cold by the mother's antibodies; he can become seriously ill from these viruses. • Infants should not be exposed to siblings or others with "a mild cold."

Doctor's Treatment

Your doctor can confirm the absence of other illnesses and complications by physical examination and sometimes will order a blood count and throat cultures. Otherwise, the course of therapy is the same as home treatment.

Related Topics: Bronchiolitis. Bronchitis. Coughs, Croup, Encephalitis. Laryngitis. Lymph Nodes—Infection Fighters. Pneumonia, Viruses

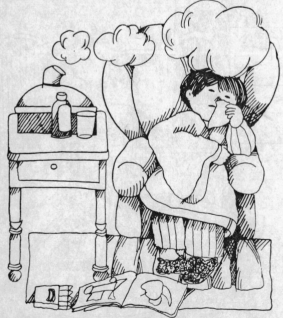

Treat the common cold with a humidifier and plenty of fluids.

CONCUSSION

Description

A concussion is an injury to the brain from a fall or blow on the head by a blunt object. In many ways a concussion is like a bruise of the brain, with swelling and sometimes escape of blood into the brain tissue. Concussions may be mild to serious.

Most children sustain one or more blows to the head during childhood. Typical reactions are immediate crying, headache, paleness, vomiting once or twice, a lump or cut at the site of injury, and sleepiness for one or two hours. These are NOT the signs of a concussion.

Signs of possible concussion are any of the following: unconsciousness at instant of injury; no memory of accident or events preceding accident; confusion (child doesn't recognize parents or know his own name); persistent vomiting; inability to walk; eyes not parallel; pupils of different sizes (Note: some children have unequal pupils normally); failure of pupils to constrict when a bright light is shined into eyes; blood coming from ear canal; bloody fluid which does not clot coming from nose; headache that continues to increase in severity; stiff neck (chin cannot be touched to chest with mouth closed); increasing drowsiness; slow pulse (less than 50 to 60 beats per minute); and abnormal breathing.

There are two rare forms of concussion in which symptoms do not develop until hours after the injury (epidural bleeding) or until days or weeks afterward (subdural bleeding).

Diagnosis

Diagnosis is made by looking for any of the symptoms listed above.

Home Treatment

Essentially, treatment of a nonpenetrating head injury is either bed rest until the child has recovered or surgery. Home treatment consists of keeping your child quiet, with his head on a pillow, and checking him frequently. He should be encouraged to sleep, but MUST be wakened every hour for evaluation of his condition until he feels well. Activity should be curtailed for at least one day after he is fully recovered. Give only aspirin or acetaminophen for headache.

Precautions

● Do not attempt home treatment if any of the above signs of concussion are present (except brief unconsciousness and lack of memory of the accident). ● Do not treat at home if scalp is depressed at the site of injury or if a gentle thumping of the skull produces the dull sound of a broken melon (these findings are rarely, if ever, present without other signs of concussion). ● Do not give pain killers, sedatives, or any medication stronger than aspirin or acetaminophen.

Doctor's Treatment

Your doctor may or may not order X rays of the skull (it is the substance of the brain that matters, not whether the skull is fractured or not), but your child may be hospitalized for observation. A CAT (computerized axial tomography) scan gives three dimensional X rays of the brain, and is most useful. Echoencephalogram, electroencephalogram, and spinal-tap tests are sometimes helpful. A consultation with a neurosurgeon may be necessary if the concussion is serious.

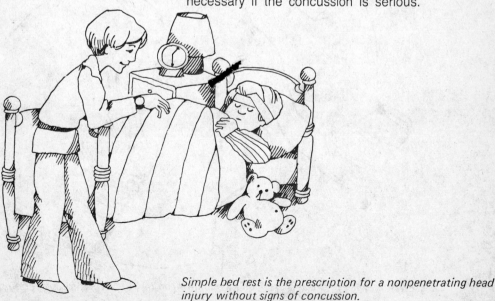

Simple bed rest is the prescription for a nonpenetrating head injury without signs of concussion.

CONJUNCTIVITIS

Description

Conjunctivitis, or pinkeye, is an infection of the transparent membrane (conjunctiva) that covers the white of the eye (sclera) and lines the undersurface of the eyelids. Conjunctivitis causes redness of the entire white of the eye and the accumulation of yellow pus. The eyelids may swell and redden, and there is a burning sensation in the eye. Vision is always normal, and light rarely bothers the eye.

Conjunctivitis is highly contagious by contact with discharge from eye or objects (e.g., hands, face cloths, toys, handkerchiefs) that have touched the infected eyes or that the child with conjunctivitis has handled. Conjunctivitis usually spreads quickly to the opposite eye.

Conjunctivitis may exist alone or as a complication of sore throat, tonsillitis, or sinusitis. The incubation period is one to three days.

Diagnosis

Conjunctivitis must be distinguished from other causes of reddened eyes. Eye allergies cause itching and tearing but never pain or pus. Viruses cause pain and tearing but no pus. Foreign bodies cause pain, sensitivity to light, tearing, no pus, and redness is usually confined to one part of the white of the eye. Glaucoma causes pain, enlargement of the pupil, tearing, and sensitivity to light but no pus. Diagnosis of conjunctivitis is a process of eliminating these other possibilities.

Home Treatment

Isolate your child. Frequently instill antibiotic eye drops or ointment into the eyes. A doctor's prescription is required, but often your doctor will oblige you by phone if your description is detailed and accurate. Treat both eyes even though only one seems involved. Continue treatment for 24 hours after the eyes appear normal. Watch other members of the family for symptoms.

Precautions

● With medication, improvement should be prompt—within 24 hours. If eyes don't clear, call your doctor. ● If eye ointments are used, there will be blurring of vision for a few minutes after each application. Any other disturbance of vision should be promptly reported to your doctor. ● Be certain to notify your doctor of any other signs of illness such as head cold, nasal discharge, sore throat, fever, or sore glands. Conjunctivitis may be part of another disease.

Doctor's Treatment

Careful examination of the outside and inside of the eyeball, including looking under the eyelids for hidden foreign bodies, are part of the doctor's treatment. Your doctor may stain the eyeball with special drops to detect injuries or ulcers and culture the eye, nasal, and throat discharge. Oral antibiotics or consultation with an ophthalmologist may be necessary.

Related Topics: Eye Allergies, Viruses

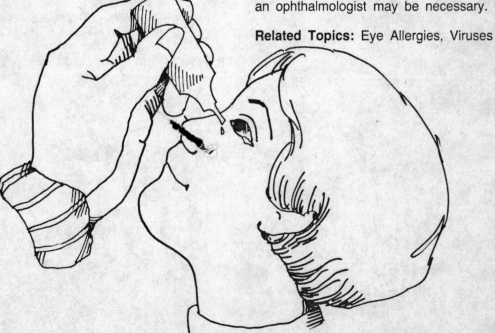

Antibiotic eye drops prescribed by a doctor can be effective in treating conjunctivitis.

Description

Constipation means that bowel movements (BMs) are too hard. Frequency is not a factor. Passage of six too-firm BMs a day is considered constipation. Passage of one BM every third or fourth day of normal or soft consistency is not constipation. Many normal, healthy children have a BM only every few days and are not constipated. The hardness of a stool is judged by appearance, by feeling, and by diameter. A stool greater than twice normal diameter must be too hard.

Constipation either has a physical, organic cause or a functional cause. Organic causes are rare and relatively easy to diagnose. They include congenital constipation (Hirschsprung's disease), which can be suspected because it starts at birth, and temporary paralysis of the intestines, seen immediately after abdominal surgery or when abdominal infections occur

Over 95 percent of constipation cases are functional and involve no physical abnormality. Functional constipation can always be cured by diet changes and daily use of stool softeners. The function of the large bowel (colon) is to store unabsorbed food waste and to absorb and conserve water from the liquid material received from the small intestine. Factors that favor the absorption of too much water by the colon lead to constipation. In children there are two common factors. The first is that the diet does not include enough roughage, which retains water. Foods that prevent constipation are: all fruits except bananas—particularly those eaten with their skin on—and fruit juices; all vegetables except peeled potatoes, especially if eaten raw; and unrefined grains and unrefined sugars (brown sugar, molasses, honey). All other foods, including milk, promote constipation. The second factor that leads to constipation is when the child resists the normal impulse to move the bowels and retains the stool. This practice permits the absorption of water by the intestine and results in stools that are too hard. The most common reason for a child's retention of the stools is his parents being overzealous in their efforts to toilet train. Passage of the too-hard stool causes pain, which reinforces the child's determination to postpone the next BM. Constipation overdistends the large bowel causing a loss of muscle tone, and the impulse to empty the bowel becomes weaker. This cycle can lead to chronic constipation. Constipation can cause pain in the anus at defecation and result in the presence of red blood on and around the BM. Other symptoms are abdominal cramps and eventual loss of appetite.

Diagnosis

Diagnosis is made by observing the character of the BM, including its diameter. However, if constipation has been present for days and weeks, paradoxical diarrhea may develop. In this condition loose, watery BMs seep around the hard stool in the colon and are passed as diarrhea. This can confuse the diagnosis.

Home Treatment

For immediate, temporary relief give an enema (disposable commerical enemas are the most convenient) or use a glycerine suppository. For a long-term permanent cure, increase the amount of roughage and decrease the amount of constipating foods in your child's diet. Since children often cannot be easily induced to eat what they should, it is often necessary to supplement their daily diet with artificial stool softeners. Stop efforts to potty train temporarily.

Precautions

● Laxatives may force passage of a hard stool and cause pain that leads to further holding back by the child. ● Enemas, suppositories, and laxatives are habit-forming.

Doctor's Treatment

Your doctor will confirm diagnosis of constipation if necessary by rectal examination and careful palpation of the child's abdomen. X-ray studies of the bowel may be required to rule out organic causes. Detailed directions and follow-up by your doctor may be necessary.

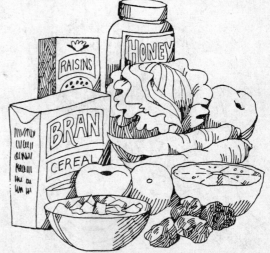

Foods that can prevent constipation are: fruits, honey, raw vegetables, and unrefined grains.

CONVULSIONS WITH FEVER

Description

Five to ten percent of all children have convulsions that are caused by fever (febrile convulsions). The speed with which the temperature rises is more crucial than its height. A sudden rise of two or three degrees may cause a seizure, but a gradual rise of five or six degrees may not.

Febrile convulsions may be likened to shaking chills that become excessive. They are most common between the ages of three months and three years. Incidence of convulsions decreases yearly from age three to age eight after which occurrence is rare. One episode of febrile convulsions usually means the child is more likely to have future ones.

During a seizure, your child will fall unconscious, become rigid, stop breathing briefly, and may turn blue. He may lose control of his bladder and stools; he may vomit. Then his limbs, torso, jaws, and eyelids will jerk convulsively, breathing will return spontaneously, and your child will recover consciousness. The entire sequence may last two to thirty minutes or longer. Your child will have no memory of the seizure. Susceptibility to febrile convulsions is not a basis on which to speculate on the likelihood of future epilepsy or brain dysfunction.

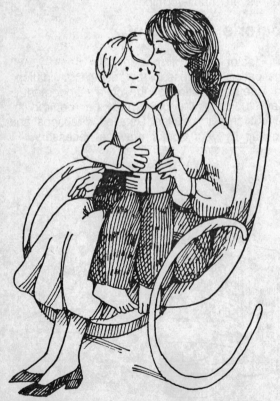

Your child will probably have no memory of a febrile convulsion.

Diagnosis

Febrile convulsions must be distinguished from convulsions caused by central nervous system disease which is accompanied by a fever but in which the disease (and not the fever) is the cause of the convulsion. These diseases include meningitis, encephalitis, and abscess of the brain. A major distinguishing characteristic of febrile convulsion is that the child recovers quickly (within minutes) and is immediately afterward alert, responsive, and not prostrated. The neck can be flexed forward after a febrile seizure ends; this is often not true with diseases involving the brain.

Home Treatment

Do not panic! Your child is in no pain and is in more danger from improper treatment than from the convulsion. Protect him from injury while the convulsion is occurring. Remove his clothing to encourage heat loss. Or wrap your child in a cool, wet sheet that has been wrung out. Give aspirin by rectal suppository if available. Notify your doctor, particularly if the convulsion lasts more than ten minutes.

Precautions

● **Do not** give aspirin or any medication by mouth to an unconscious child. ● Do not give artificial respiration. Muscles of respiration are temporarily in spasm and forceful artificial respiration may be injurious. ● Placing a convulsing child in a tub of water may reduce temperature, but accidents such as scalding and injuries against the sides of the tub have resulted; this practice is NOT recommended.

Doctor's Treatment

Your doctor may give an anticonvulsant—usually phenobarbital or diazepam by injection—and do a complete physical examination, taking blood tests and a spinal tap to confirm diagnosis. Anticonvulsants may be recommended for future fevers. If the febrile convulsion is atypical or recurrent your doctor may order additional tests such as an electroencephalogram, echoencephalogram, and CAT (computerized axial tomography) scan. Daily anticonvulsants are prescribed for several years under some circumstances.

Related Topics: Convulsions without Fever, Fever, Encephalitis, Meningitis

CONVULSIONS WITHOUT FEVER

Description

Convulsions without fever (also known as epilepsy or recurrent seizures) generally occur at a later age than febrile convulsions, but they may start in infancy. Several patterns of seizures exist. The most common resembles a febrile convulsion and is called a major (grand mal) seizure. It is characterized by an abrupt onset of unconsciousness and a stiffening of the limbs and trunk followed by generalized jerking and recovery. A major seizure may be preceded by a warning sensation (aura) and your child may cry out at the onset. Your child usually will be confused and sleepy after the seizure ends.

Less common types of convulsions without fever are momentary periods of unconsciousness that last for a few seconds with minimal muscular activity such as: nodding of head; fluttering of eyes (petit mal); localized convulsions involving only parts of the body (Jacksonian seizures); and convulsions that cause only changes in behavior and personality of a periodic nature (psychomotor seizures). Most of these types of epilepsy have no discoverable cause. Causes of nonepileptic, recurrent seizures are kidney failure, disturbances of calcium metabolism, liver failure, low blood sugar, degenerative diseases, and injuries to the brain.

Diagnosis

Diagnosis cannot be made without laboratory tests and a neurological examination.

Home Treatment

The most important thing is to prevent your child from injury during the thrashing phase of convulsion. Your child may bite his tongue during the attack; if possible put a soft object such as a folded handkerchief between the back teeth on one side. Do not put your fingers in the child's mouth. Until the seizures are controlled (which may take years), safeguard your child from possible serious injury provoked by seizure by discouraging him from climbing high ladders or tall trees; do not allow him to swim alone. Otherwise, your child can and should live a completely normal life with unrestricted activities.

Precautions

● Do not assume that your child has been made unconscious by a fall. Do consider the possibility that epilepsy has led to a fall and unconsciousness.

Doctor's Treatment

Your doctor will perform physical and neurological examinations, an electroencephalogram, a skull X ray, an echoencephalogram, a CAT (computerized axial tomography) scan, a determination of blood chemistries, and possibly a spinal tap. A wide assortment of potent anticonvulsant medications are available by prescription. These drugs may be prescribed for daily use for many years. Guidance in dosage can be obtained by blood tests. In difficult cases, your doctor may recommend consultation with a neurologist.

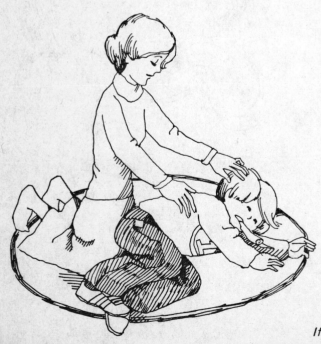

If your child has a convulsion, try to protect him from injury.

COUGHS

Description

Coughing is a valuable defense mechanism that guards the respiratory tree against foreign material. Not a disease itself, coughing is a reflex that is set off by any foreign matter that has entered or seeks to enter the respiratory tree and by any irritation of the lining of the tree. (The respiratory tree includes the throat, larynx, trachea, bronchial tubes, and lungs.) Most often, coughing is beneficial, but sometimes it is ineffective. The chief harm it can produce is interference with sleep and exhaustion from muscular effort. Coughing also may lead to vomiting, and in young infants if it is severe and prolonged enough, injury of the bronchial tree may result.

Most coughs are caused by viruses (common colds, croup, bronchitis, bronchiolitis). Some are caused by bacteria (sinusitis, epiglottitis, bacterial pneumonia, pertussis), some by allergies (asthma), and some by inhaled foreign bodies.

Diagnosis

A cough is only as serious as the disease or condition that causes it. As with a fever, a child with a cough is no less ill if you suppress the cough. A child with a mild illness and a cough is still only mildly ill. To correct the cough, cure the disease. (See the Chart of Symptoms at the front of this book to pinpoint the diseases for which coughing is a symptom.)

Home Treatment

Cough medicines are intended to: reduce the frequency of the cough by suppressing the cough reflex; loosen a tight cough; dry up a loose cough; or combat an allergy responsible for coughing. They often contain ingredients to accomplish more than one of these goals at the same time. Before purchasing a cough medicine for home use, determine which of the four goals listed above you want accomplished. Cough *suppressants* contain a narcotic (codeine, dihydrocodeinone, or hydromorphine) or a nonnarcotic (dextromethorphan, or benzonatate). Consult your doctor about using a narcotic cough suppressant. *Cough looseners* contain an expectorant (glyceryl-guaiacolate, guaifenesin, ammonium chloride, or antimony potassium tartrate). *Cough tighteners* contain a decongestant (ephedrine, pseudoephedrine, phenyl-propanolamine, or homatropine), and *antiallergy drugs* contain ephedrine or an antihistamine.

Virtually all combinations of the above drugs are on the market in liquid form or as tablets or capsules. Although not generally thought of as cough medicines but valuable for allergic coughs are the antiasthma medications aminophylline, theophylline, and metaproterenol.

Precautions

● Do not give cough medicine to a child with croup. ● Do not give cough medicines to a child with breathing difficulty unless you know you are treating asthma; give only antiasthma drugs. ● Do not give cough medicines to a child who may have inhaled a foreign body.

Doctor's Treatment

Your doctor will direct treatment toward the condition causing the cough not at the cough itself. Narcotic cough medicines and some with antihistamines require a doctor's prescription.

Related Topics: Asthma, Bronchiolitis, Bronchitis, Common Cold, Croup

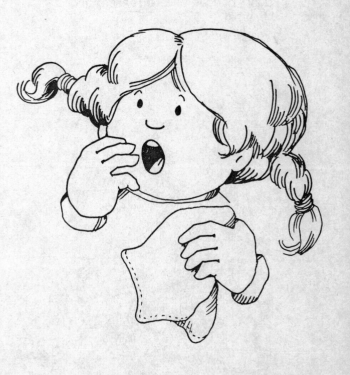

Coughing is a protective reflex.

Description

Cradle cap (seborrheic dermatitis) consists of adherent yellowish, scaly or crusted patches on the scalp, composed largely of oil and dead cells. It is most common in infants but is seen in children through age five. The disease may extend onto the forehead and may also be present in the skin fold behind the ears, on the ears, and in the diaper area. The most typical location is over the anterior fontanelle (the soft spot). Temporary loss of hair is common.

Diagnosis

Diagnosis can be made from the locations and appearance of the patches and by the greasy scalp film that can be scraped off.

Home Treatment

Mild cases of cradle cap on the scalp can be cured by daily, vigorous shampooing using soap on a wet, rough facecloth wrapped around the palm of your hand. Special shampoos that contain coal tar or salicylic acid are useful. Apply ointments containing sulfur, salicylic acid, or coal tar to the scalp and other areas daily.

Precautions

● Be sure that medicated shampoos and ointments do not get into your child's eyes.
● Discontinue using these preparations if irritation and reddening of the scalp or skin occur.

Doctor's Treatment

Your doctor will confirm diagnosis by differentiating cradle cap from eczema, yeast infections, and contact dermatitis. The doctor's treatment will be the same as home treatment. In addition a steroid cream or ointment may be prescribed.

Related Topic: Eczema

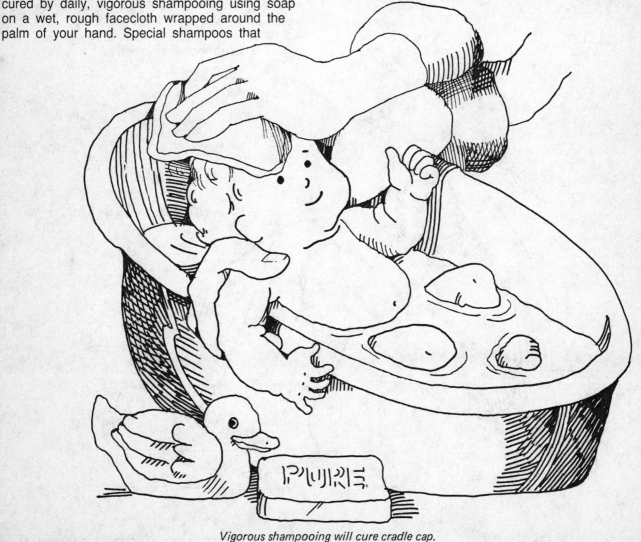

Vigorous shampooing will cure cradle cap.

CREEPING ERUPTION

Description

Cutaneous larvae migrans, popularly known as creeping eruption, is an infestation of the skin caused by hookworm larvae from a cat or dog. It is usually contracted through the sand or dirt in which an animal has defecated. The condition is common along the Atlantic Coast (south from Virginia), in Florida, and along the Gulf Coast.

The microscopic larvae penetrate the skin and burrow just beneath the surface forming erratic, wavy, red ink-like lines several inches long. The usual areas involved are the buttocks, feet, and hands, but creeping eruption may appear anywhere on the skin.

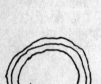

Diagnosis

Diagnosis is made by observing the typical, wandering, red lines, which are usually the width of a pen stroke.

Home Treatment

Creeping eruption used to be treated by freezing larva at the end of the burrow with ethyl chloride. A doctor's treatment is preferred and recommended.

Precautions

● Do not allow children to go barefooted in areas contaminated by cat and dog feces. ● If ethyl chloride spray is used, care must be taken to avoid freezing the skin and producing chilblains and frostbite.

Doctor's Treatment

Treatment is with thiabendazole (an antiworm medicine available by prescription only). Medication is given orally twice daily for two days. The treatment may have to be repeated.

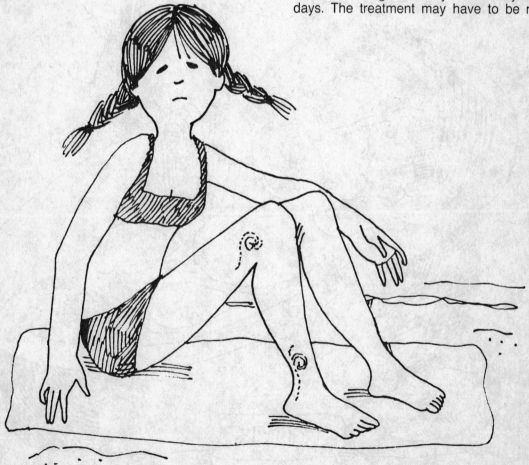

Creeping eruption causes characteristic wandering red lines to appear on the skin. Treatment by a doctor is recommended.

Description

The eyeballs are turned in all directions by six tiny (extraocular) muscles that lie within the bony socket. These muscles keep the eyes parallel when the child looks at a distant object (more than 20 feet) and slightly converge the eyes when they are focusing on closer objects.

Infants learn to focus their eyes during their first three to six months. Occasionally, their eyes turn in (esotropia, internal strabismus) or out (exotropia, external strabismus) in relation to each other. These conditions may briefly occur even up to age one and still be considered normal. When an infant's eyes are continuously not parallel, when they are not parallel with increasing frequency at any age, or when they are not parallel past age one, the situation is abnormal and requires your doctor's advice.

Most cases of crossed eyes result from improper functioning of the extraocular muscles. Some are caused by a visual defect in one or both eyes. Anything that can cause strabismus can also cause the development of a "lazy eye" (amblyopia ex anopsia). If this condition is not corrected by age seven, loss of sight due to disuse may result.

Diagnosis

Diagnosis is made by observing the relationship of the eyes to each other as the child focuses near and far and looks to either side and up and down.

Most strabismus reported by parents is an optical illusion, and the child's eyes are actually straight. Many infants and young children have an extra skinfold at the nasal side of the eyelids, present because of the tininess of the bridge of the nose (epicanthal fold). This extra fold allows more of the white of the eye to show toward the temples than toward the nose, creating an illusion of crossed eyes. Straightness of the eyes is best judged by observing the position of the reflected points of light in both eyes (highlights). Identical location of the highlights in both eyes proves eyes are parallel.

Home Treatment

There is no home treatment except under supervision and instruction by your doctor.

Precautions

● If the pupils of your child's eyes are not equally black, smoothly round, and the same size, report to your doctor. ● If your child's eyes are not parallel, see your doctor to avoid amblyopia. ● Visual acuity (sharpness of vision) should be checked annually in all children from age three.

Doctor's Treatment

Your doctor will check extraocular muscles and vision and inspect the inside of the eyeballs. This examination can be done on any child at any age. If diagnosis of crossed eyes is confirmed, treatment will depend upon the cause. It may include eye surgery, glasses, patching of one eye, daily use of eye drops, or eye muscle exercises guided by a specialist. If strabismus is diagnosed or suspected, your doctor will probably recommend that you consult an ophthalmologist (a physician who specializes in eyes.)

Related Topic: Lazy Eye

Crossed eyes, a weakness of eye muscles which causes the eyeballs to converge more than they should, cannot be treated at home without specific instructions from a doctor.

CROUP

Description

Croup is a common, contagious illness of children contracted in the same manner as a common cold—by airborne droplets and direct contact with an infected person. Croup is characterized by a tight, dry, barking cough and by hoarseness. Difficult breathing develops quickly with more pronounced trouble breathing *in* than breathing *out*. This is the opposite of that seen in asthma. Efforts to breathe in cause the typical crowing sound associated with croup.

Basically, there are three types of croup: diphtheria, spasmodic croup, and epiglottitis. *Spasmodic croup* is common and is usually caused by a virus (parainfluenza, adenoviruses, syncytial virus, or influenza). Spasmodic croup most often occurs between three months and three years of age and represents an infection of the vocal cords and voice box (larynx). It is similar to laryngitis in the adolescent or adult. Fever is absent or low-grade (101°F). The disease may occur once in a child, or repeatedly with every head cold. Children who experience recurrent croup often develop other forms of respiratory allergies later. Spasmodic croup can be serious, but milder cases, especially recurrent ones, can be safely handled at home.

Epiglottitis is a severe, rapidly progressive, **life-threatening illness**—a true emergency in which minutes count. It is an infection of the epiglottis (covering of the larynx) and adjacent tissues caused by bacteria. Epiglottitis has all the symptoms of spasmodic croup. It is most common in children between three and nine years of age. There is also a rising fever from 103°F to 105°F. Difficulty with breathing increases progressively and your child may have trouble swallowing, preferring to sit with his head forward, mouth open, and tongue partially out. The condition rapidly progresses to choking, convulsions, and death if untreated.

Diagnosis

The combination of a barking cough, hoarseness, difficult breathing and a crowing sound on inhalation is obvious croup. For all practical purposes, diphtheria can be ruled out as a cause if your child has been properly immunized. Choking on an aspirated foreign object may resemble croup but can also be ruled out by history, fever (if present), and the ability of the child to talk.

In epiglottitis a definitive diagnostic sign is the appearance of a swollen, red epiglottis at the base of the tongue. (Use a flashlight to look, but **do not depress the tongue** in an effort to see the epiglottis as this may cause instant and complete obstruction of the air passage.)

It is important always to consider the possibility of epiglottitis as a cause of croup when any of the above symptoms are present.

Home Treatment

Use steam from a vaporizer or humidifier. Steam also may be generated quickly and temporarily by running a hot shower in a closed bathroom. Sit in the room with your child for a short while. In spasmodic croup, especially without fever. a single, large, oral dose of a steroid, given with your doctor's permission, can be miraculous, giving relief in 15 minutes. Unless you have witnessed croup before, it is best to consult your doctor with first attack.

Precautions

● Ipecac as a home treatment for croup is no longer recommended since its use may depress respiration. ● Never give suppressant cough medicines to a child with croup. ● If you suspect epiglottitis, notify your doctor and head for the nearest hospital emergency room.

Doctor's Treatment

For spasmodic croup your doctor's treatment will be the same as your home treatment. However, the doctor may hospitalize your child and use a croup tent with high humidity, order cultures and blood count, prescribe antibiotics, and use isoproterenol by inhalation. If the condition becomes severe your doctor may have to perform a tracheostomy.

Epiglottitis is always treated as an emergency. Your child may be intubated (have a tube inserted in his airway). If necessary, a tracheostomy is performed, intravenous fluids and antibiotics are given, and the child is monitored.

Related Topics: Choking, Diphtheria

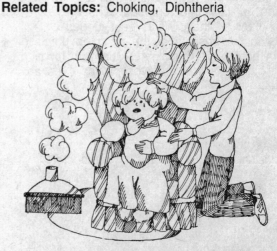

Steam from a vaporizer is helpful in treating croup.

CUTS

Description

Wounds of the skin are classified as abrasions (scrapes), punctures, and lacerations. A laceration is a cut of any size and depth and can be located anywhere on the body. Major lacerations obviously need a doctor's immediate attention; emergency control of bleeding is the only necessary home treatment.

Some smaller cuts can be tended as well at home as by a doctor; some cannot. If a cut is more than skin deep it cannot be treated at home. Deeper structures, such as muscles, tendons, nerves, and deeper layers of the scalp, must be repaired by sewing. A laceration with ragged edges or one that is deeply embedded with dirt needs professional care to avoid infection and to minimize scarring.

A cut heals leaving a scar the size of the opening of the skin. No treatment will reduce the length of a cut or resulting scar, but the closer the edges of the cut are to one another during the healing process, the narrower the final scar. If the edges of the cut can be held together by bandaging at home there may be no advantage to a doctor's treatment. However, if the cut involves an area that moves, such as that near a joint or parts of the face, it is virtually impossible to keep the edges from gaping without the wound being sewn. A small cut rarely requires suturing to control the bleeding.

Diagnosis

Whether a cut needs a doctor's care depends upon careful inspection after the bleeding has stopped. You must evaluate the width and depth, the dirtiness and raggedness, and whether a home-style bandage can hold the edges together for the seven to ten days required for healing.

Home Treatment

First, stop the bleeding by applying firm pressure directly on the cut for ten minutes (by the clock). Use sterile gauze if it's immediately available, but any reasonably clean cloth—a handkerchief, towel, or shirt—will do. Even bleeding from large arteries can be controlled by pressure; you never need so-called pressure points. Only if a limb is partially or completely amputated will a tourniquet be necessary, and then it may be applied anywhere above the wound. (A tourniquet seldom if ever needs to be used. The new thinking is that once put on, it should be left on, not released and tightened as instructions once indicated. Patient should be rushed to a medical facility with no delay!)

Second, once the bleeding has stopped, wash the area with soap and water so that the cut is clearly visible. If home treatment appears reasonable apply a nonstinging antiseptic and draw the wound's edges together with adhesive butterflies or Steristrips bandages (both available at your pharmacy). Cuts near the joints of your child's fingers can be immobilized by splinting the fingers till the cut has healed. Cuts between the toes can sometimes be immobilized by bandaging adjacent toes together. Cover the wound with sterile dressing, inspect it every day for infection, and remove butterflies or Steristrips bandages after seven to ten days.

Precautions

● If the laceration requires sewing it must be done within eight hours to avoid infection. ● If the home-treated wound becomes infected (showing increased tenderness, swelling, discharge of pus, or red streaks radiating from wound) see your doctor. ● Be sure that tetanus immunization is current.

Doctor's Treatment

A doctor, surgeon, or plastic surgeon has facilities and skill to handle cuts that are beyond home care.

Related Topics: Immunizations, Puncture Wounds, Scrapes

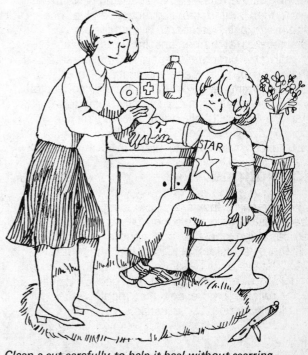

Clean a cut carefully to help it heal without scarring.

CYSTIC FIBROSIS

Description

Cystic fibrosis is a chronic, inherited disease which affects the lungs, pancreas, sweat glands, and sometimes the liver and other organs. Five percent of Caucasians, two percent of American blacks, and less than one percent of Orientals and native African blacks are healthy carriers. One in 2,000 Caucasian children has CF and 25 percent of offspring of parents who are both carriers may be affected.

CF may be present at birth as complete intestinal obstruction. In infancy and childhood common symptoms are: recurrent respiratory infections including bronchitis and pneumonia; chronic cough; failure to gain adequate weight; constipation or diarrhea with foul stools; prolapse of the rectum, and clubbing (broadening) of the fingertips and toes. Sometimes symptoms are not apparent until school age or adolescence.

Diagnosis

Diagnosis is confirmed by a specific, inexpensive test called "the sweat test." Sometimes CF is suspected by the appearance of a chest X ray or by the very salty taste of a child's sweat when kissed. The earlier the diagnosis is made and treatment started, the more favorable the outcome.

Home Treatment

Home treatment is extensive and important but only under your doctor's direction and advice. Treatment lasts for years, is usually administered at home; and includes antibiotics, special diet, pancreatic enzymes by mouth, inhalations of vapor and medications, and postural drainage. (Postural drainage, conducted in a home setting, involves positioning the child over the bed with his head pillowed on the floor. The child's chest is tapped soundly to allow excessive fluids to drain from the lungs.

Precautions

● If your child shows any CF symptoms, a sweat test should be done. It is painless, harmless, inexpensive, and generally reliable. ● If there is history of CF in the family, a sweat test should be done on all children, even though they appear healthy. ● The sweat test is not reliable before age one month and is not as reliable during adolescence.

Doctor's Treatment

If the diagnosis of CF is established, your doctor will refer you to a medical center where there are specialists in treating CF. Sometimes surgery is necessary. The outlook for prolonged life of a child with CF who is in relatively good health is better now than in the past, but a cure for CF is still being sought.

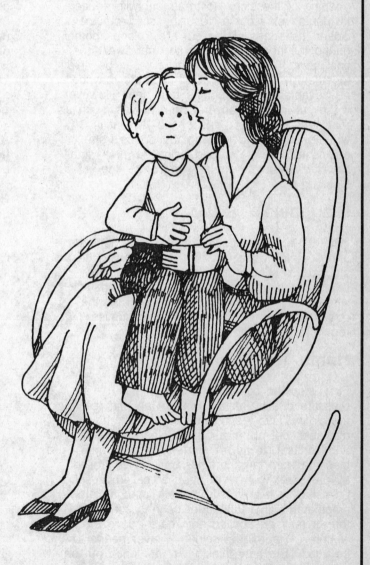

The very salty taste of a child's sweat might be a sign of CF. Professional diagnosis involves a "sweat test."

Description

Normal hearing depends upon sound waves passing down the ear canal and setting the eardrum to vibrating: that, in turn, moves the three tiny bones in the middle ear. This motion is transmitted across the middle ear to the inner ear (cochlea), where the vibrations are changed to electrical impulses which are carried to the brain via the eighth cranial nerve and are interpreted as sound by the brain. Damage, disease, or malfunction of any of these structures can result in deafness.

A hearing loss may be slight or severe. It may involve one or both ears and may be present at birth or develop at any age. Any of the following problems can lead to hearing difficulties.

Ear canal problems: impacted wax, foreign body in canal, swimmer's ear (otitis externa);

Drum and middle ear problems: abscessed ear (otitis media), obstructed eustachean tube (the tube that connects the nose and the middle ear);

Inner ear problems: infections, usually viral, or caused by an injury;

Eighth cranial nerve problems: this nerve may be nonfunctioning at birth (congenital deafness or intrauterine infection with rubella virus), damaged after birth by injury or by infection with virus (mumps, measles), bacteria (meningitis), or by medications (streptomycin, kanamycin, gentamicin, polymyxin, and neomycin).

Diagnosis

Suspect hearing loss if any of the following symptoms are observed: your infant over three months old ignores sounds or does not turn head toward sound; your baby over one year old does not speak at least a few words; your child over two years old does not speak in at least two- to three-word sentences; your child over five years old does not speak so that a stranger can understand him; your child has learning problems in school at any age; or your child does not appear to hear well at home. Any of these symptoms may be caused by hearing loss, but they also may be the result of other causes.

Home Treatment

Treatment depends upon the cause, as well as upon the degree of the hearing loss. If the problem seems to be earwax the use of Debrox eardrops for several nights will often aid in wax removal. (Some doctor's recommend that the ear be flushed with water from a syringe; there is a risk to this procedure, however.) If the child has a head cold, the hearing loss is apt to be due to obstruction of the eustachian tube. If there is no earache the cold symptoms can be treated with nose drops and an oral decongestant.

Precautions

● If you are a woman of child-bearing age consult your doctor about rubella immunization. A simple blood test will determine whether or not you've been immunized. ● Do not put any object, including cotton swabs, into your child's ear canal for any reason. You may impact the wax or damage the drum.

Doctor's Treatment

Your doctor will examine the ear to determine the cause of deafness. Hearing can be tested by specialists in children of any age past early infancy by various devices and instruments. There are federally funded speech and hearing centers in all states to which a doctor can refer your child if diagnosis, cause, or treatment of hearing loss is in doubt. Your deaf child should start special education as soon as the condition is discovered, even if he is as young as one or two years old.

Related Topics: Draining Ear, Earaches, Immunizations, Swimmer's Ear

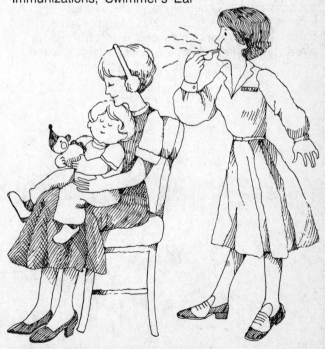

Hearing specialists can easily test the hearing ability of any child past early infancy.

DEHYDRATION

Description

Dehydration means drying out. It is caused by the loss of fluids from the body in excess of the amount of fluids taken in. In addition to the loss of water, dehydration is accompanied by the loss of minerals and salts from the body. Fluids, minerals, and salts are lost from the body through diarrhea, vomiting and sweating, through water vapor from the lungs with excessive breathing (as in bronchiolitis and asthma), and in the urine (in diabetes). The quantity of water in the body and the proper concentration of salts and minerals are vital to health and to life.

The smaller the child the more quickly dehydration can develop. In young infants dehydration occurs as rapidly as 12 to 24 hours from onset of one of the above causes. Dehydration as a result of diminished intake of liquids in a child who is not losing fluids from some other cause is rare. Except in young infants and in children with diabetes, the kidneys can compensate for small fluid intake. But a diminished intake of liquids in a child who is also losing fluids hastens dehydration.

Diagnosis

Except in the presence of diabetes, dehydration can be detected by observing the urinary output. A young child who goes six to eight hours without urinating and an older child who does not urinate for ten to twelve hours may be dehydrated. Other signs of dehydration include: sunken eyes; dryness (to an exploring finger) of the membranes of the mouth; loss of elasticity of the skin when pinched between the thumb and forefinger; drowsiness; rapid or slow breathing; and depression of the soft spot in an infant.

Home Treatment

Vomiting, if present, must be stopped. With any condition that causes fluid loss—including prolonged high fever—you should encourage your child to drink extra fluids. The best liquids to give a child with a severe case of dehydration are commercial fluids that contain proper salts and sugar (Lytren and Pedialyte mineral and electrolyte mixtures). Other good liquids are gelatin desserts (liquid or jelled), weak tea with sugar, ginger ale, colas and other carbonated drinks, and fruit juices. Plain water is less helpful. Whole milk and skimmed milk diluted by a half with water are sometimes tolerated.

Precautions

● **Undiluted skimmed milk and boiled whole milk are forbidden** because the salt and mineral content is too great for the child to tolerate. ● If symptoms of dehydration develop, contact your doctor; the younger the child the more urgent the situation. ● Urinary output is totally unreliable in judging dehydration in a diabetic.

Doctor's Treatment

Your doctor will diagnose and treat the underlying condition. Your child may be admitted to a hospital for intravenous fluids and salts and for tests to detect salt and mineral disturbances.

Related Topics: Asthma, Bronchiolitis, Diabetes, Diarrhea, Fever, Vomiting

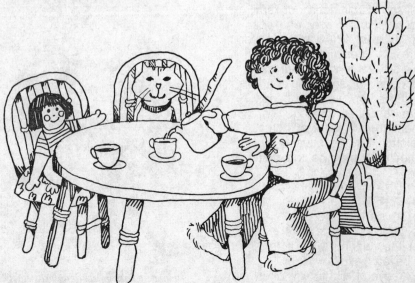

To compensate for any condition that causes the loss of fluids, encourage your child to drink extra liquids.

DIABETES

Description

Diabetes is a condition of altered metabolism caused by the insufficient production of insulin by the pancreas. The most obvious metabolic change is the impaired utilization of sugars (and starches), resulting in elevated blood sugar, the passage of sugar in the urine, and the burning of fats in place of sugar. This disease process produces toxic substances called ketone bodies in the body and urine.

Diabetes can occur at any age. It is present in one in 2,500 children by age 15 years. The disease is generally transmitted genetically through both parents, who may or may not be diabetic.

The earliest signs of diabetes are an increase in hunger, urination (both in frequency and in total quantity), and thirst. Weight loss, fatigue, and irritability follow. Most cases are detected by this stage. If not detected and corrected, deep, rapid breathing and unconsciousness (diabetic coma) eventually develop.

Diagnosis

The symptoms of diabetes can give the first indication of the disease at home. The definitive diagnosis is made only by laboratory tests—a urinalysis shows presence of sugar and ketone bodies, and a blood test shows elevated blood sugar. A glucose tolerance test also may be required in which the child drinks a known amount of glucose sugar, and the blood sugar level is measured periodically for several hours.

Home Treatment

Treatment is tailored to your child's exact needs by your doctor. You and your child must become thoroughly knowledgeable about diabetes—dietary restrictions, administration of insulin, periodic testing of urine, and the recognition and treatment of insulin shock.

Precautions

● Bedwetting that begins to occur regularly after your child has been night-trained for some time can indicate developing diabetes. Have the urine tested for diabetes (and infection) if bedwetting persists. ● If there is diabetes in your family's background, guard against obesity in your children. Being overweight makes a child who is already predisposed to diabetes more susceptible to its developing beyond the latent stage as he grows older. ● Because the sugar in the urine prevents the kidneys from conserving the body's fluids, untreated and uncontrolled diabetes may lead to dehydration. Complicating this situation is the fact that a decrease in urination is not a reliable sign of dehydration in diabetes.

Doctor's Treatment

Your doctor will initially hospitalize your child to regulate his diet and insulin requirements and to combat dehydration and ketosis if present. Before discharging your child, your doctor will make certain that you and the child are knowledgeable about administration of insulin and regulation of diet. Most diabetic children require insulin daily and are instructed—from as early as four years of age—to give themselves injections.

Related Topic: Dehydration

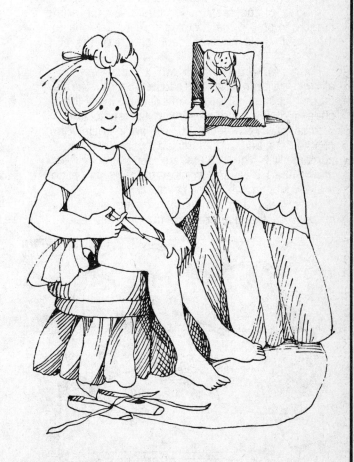

Diabetic children can learn to give themselves insulin injections.

DIAPER RASHES

Description

Rashes in the diaper area may be due to the chemicals used in washing cloth diapers—detergent, bleach, whitener, water-softener, or soap—or to the chemicals used in the manufacture of disposable diapers. Diaper rashes are red, slightly rough and scaly, and distributed over the total area touched by the diapers. A variant of diaper rash is caused by the plastic outer layer of the disposable diapers or by the plastic or rubber pants worn over cloth diapers. Other rashes in this area include:

Ammonia rash, in which the skin is burned by ammonia from urine decomposed by normal bacteria of the skin. This condition is worse after long sleep. It is identified by an ammonia smell when changing the diaper;

Yeast rash, which is common during the first weeks of life and after the child has been given antibiotics. The rash is composed of countless red, scaly spots, each several pinheads in size and representing a colony of yeast. The spots may all run together into a solid area, but identifiable islands are present at the edge of the rash. It is caused by the same fungus (monilia) that causes thrush. Lesions in the mouth help confirm identification of the rash;

Food and drug rashes, which occur in allergic children and are caused by new foods or medications. There is often a rash on the cheeks of the face present at the same time;

Infectious rashes, which are an infantile form of impetigo and are identified by blisters that contain pus. The blisters are generally match-head size and smaller than the impetigo that occurs in the older child;

Seborrhea, a common rash in the skin creases of the diaper area. It is usually accompanied by seborrhea elsewhere such as on the scalp (cradle cap) and behind the ears; and

Contagious disease rashes such as the rashes that accompany chicken pox, measles, and scarlet fever. Sometimes the rash appears in the diaper area a day before it spreads to more typical areas.

Diagnosis

Diagnosis depends upon history—a recent change to different diapers or the manner of laundering them, new foods, or treatment with antibiotics—appearance and location of rash, presence of ammonia odor, and the presence of lesions elsewhere on the body.

Home Treatment

Change soap brands or the method of washing the diapers. Apply protective ointments (petroleum jelly, zinc oxide, vitamin A & D ointment, or Desitin ointment). For rash from ammonia use anti-ammoniacal powders and ointments. Avoid airtight outer covering over diapers. If rash is severe, your doctor can prescribe oral medications. For rash from yeast see Thrush. For rash from foods and drugs eliminate new foods, beverages, and medicines started in the past month. Apply steroid preparations locally. Then re-introduce stopped foods one at a time at weekly intervals in order to determine the offender. For rash from infections wash with soap and water and apply antibiotic ointment (bacitracin, neomycin) frequently. If rash is spreading or severe or if it is accompanied by fever, irritability, or loss of appetite see your doctor.

Precautions

● If the rash gets worse even after two days of home treatment, reassess your diagnosis or see your doctor. ● Do not use ointments in combination (those that contain an antibiotic, fungicide, and steroid) without your doctor's approval. ● If your child has any other symptoms see your doctor.

Doctor's Treatment

Your doctor will identify a rash by appearance and history and may culture or scrape rash for identification of bacteria or funguses. Oral antibiotics or medicated ointment may be prescribed for diagnostic/therapeutic trial.

Related Topics: Cradle Cap, Eczema, Thrush

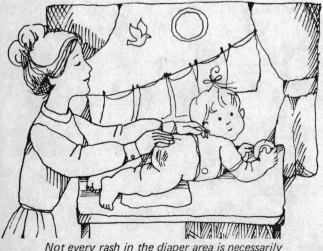

Not every rash in the diaper area is necessarily diaper rash.

DIARRHEA/CHILDREN

Description

As in infants, diarrhea in children refers to the looseness of the stools and not to the frequency of bowel movements (BMs). The number of BMs per day measures the severity of the diarrhea. The condition in children over the age of five differs in several respects from that which occurs in infants. The likelihood of dehydration decreases with the increasing age and size of the child. Serious dehydration is unlikely past six years old unless diarrhea is accompanied by vomiting that interferes with liquid intake. Enteric viruses (those in the intestine) are the most common cause of diarrhea in older children, followed by dysentery bacteria and intestinal parasites. Respiratory viruses and food intolerances are the least likely cause of this condition in older children. Other causes of diarrhea, which are rare or unknown in infants but prevalent in older children and which can produce prolonged and recurrent illness, include ulcerative colitis and regional enteritis (Crohn's disease) —inflammatory diseases of unestablished cause.

Diagnosis

As in infants, the diagnosis depends upon character of the stool and upon the child's history.

Home Treatment

If present, treat vomiting first. Limit or eliminate solids, especially those with roughage, fruits (except bananas), vegetables, butter and fatty meats, and peanut butter. Eliminate milk since diarrhea often causes temporary intolerance to milk which further aggravates diarrhea. Encourage clear liquids.

Kaolin and pectin mixtures may slow diarrhea, but do little for cramps. Consult your doctor about using anti-diarrheal remedies. Paregoric and tablets or liquid containing diphenoxylate (for older children) may stop cramps and lessen diarrhea. Hyoscyamine, atropine, and hyoscine preparations also reduce cramps. These anti-diarrheal remedies are available at your pharmacy. (Kaolin and pectin are the only OTC preparations.)

Precautions

● Isolate an infant from siblings who are ill with vomiting and diarrhea. ● Report blood in stools, high fever, prostration, severe or prolonged (more than two to three days) diarrhea to your doctor; dysentery may be the cause. ● Report frequently recurrent diarrhea to your doctor since the diarrhea may be a symptom of colitis or enteritis, especially if there is weight loss.

Doctor's Treatment

Your doctor's treatment will be the same as home treatment. Blood tests, X rays of large and small bowels, sigmoidoscopy, intestinal antibiotics, and steroids also may be necessary. In severe cases, hospitalization may be ordered.

Related Topics: Constipation, Dehydration, Diarrhea/Infants, Dysentery, Vomiting

Intestinal viruses are the most common cause of diarrhea in children over the age of five

DIARRHEA/INFANTS

Description

Diarrhea refers to the consistency of the stool and not to the frequency of bowel movements (BMs). Any BM that is partially or completely runny constitutes diarrhea. The loose and watery stools often contain mucus and sometimes flecks of red blood, and BMs number from one to twenty per day. (The frequency and volume of the loose stools is a measure of the severity of the diarrhea.) Diarrhea may be accompanied by cramps and sometimes fever, loss of appetite, vomiting, and weight loss. The condition in infants and young children is potentially dangerous because of the increased likelihood of dehydration.

The usual causes of diarrhea are infections of the digestive tract and intolerance to foods. In infants, infections may be caused by respiratory viruses as well as intestinal viruses, bacteria (coliform and dysentary bacilli, staph), and parasites (Giardia, amebae). Two examples of foods which may be inherently improper for infants in general are corn kernels or large quantities of prunes. Other foods may be wrong

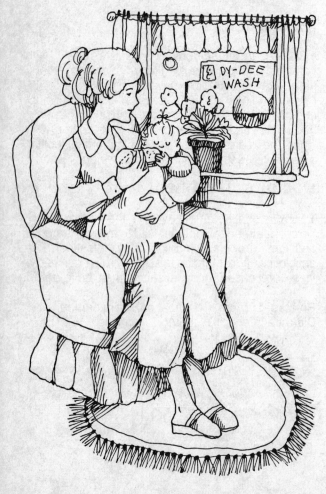

Diarrhea in infants can lead to dehydration.

for a particular infant with food intolerances or allergies. Many antibiotics also may cause diarrhea in infants.

Diagnosis

The character of the stools is definitive. One or two loose BMs followed by a return to normal do not represent a significant case of diarrhea. The cause of diarrhea may be suggested by the foods recently added to the infant's diet, cases in older siblings, or recent antibiotic therapy.

Home Treatment

If present, vomiting must be treated first. Eliminate all newly introduced foods and beverages. If diarrhea is mild, eliminate foods with roughage. Stop all fruits (except bananas) and vegetables and minimize fruit juices. If diarrhea is mild, dilute milk by half with water; if diarrhea is severe, eliminate all solids and milk altogether. Encourage the child to drink liquids to ward off dehydration.

There exists sharp disagreement among children's doctors about the safety of anti-diarrheal medications. Mixtures of kaolin and pectin, with or without paregoric, or a prescription of sulfonamide and tincture of opium may be tried, but check with your doctor first.

Precautions

● Continue treatment until there is no stool or normal stools for 24 to 48 hours. ● Solids aggravate diarrhea and can be avoided for many days without any danger to general health. Liquid intake is of paramount importance. ● Watch for symptoms of dehydration. ● Improperly prepared and refrigerated formulas are a common cause of serious infant diarrhea, especially under primitive conditions of sanitation (camping and traveling).

Doctor's Treatment

Your doctor's procedure will be the same as your home treatment but your doctor may want to evaluate the seriousness of dehydration. (The loss of ten percent of a baby's weight indicates serious dehydration.) Stools may be cultured for bacteria. Hospitalization may be required for administration of intravenous fluids and for investigation of a possible malabsorption problem.

Related Topics: Constipation, Dehydration, Diarrhea/Children, Dysentery, Intestinal Allergies, Viruses, Vomiting

DIPHTHERIA

Description

Diphtheria is a frequently fatal disease caused by a specific bacterium, Corynebacterium diphtheriae, and caught by exposure to a person with the disease or to a carrier of the disease. The germ causes infection of the nose, throat, tonsils, and lymph nodes of the neck. The microorganism kills, sometimes by destroying tissue, and sometimes by producing a toxin that causes heart damage and paralysis. The incubation period is two to four days. The infected throat develops pus and a gray membrane that looks similar to strep throat and mononucleosis. Croup and pneumonia are common complications.

The protective immunization against diphtheria has been available for over 40 years and is among the safest, cheapest, and most effective of all known vaccines. Despite the availability of the vaccine, diphtheria still exists throughout the world.

Diagnosis

Diphtheria is difficult to diagnose for three reasons: First, many American doctors have never seen a case in training or practice. Second, diphtheria closely resembles mononucleosis, strep throat, and other forms of croup. And finally, routine throat cultures taken in a doctor's office for detection of strep do not show diphtheria bacilli. (Twenty percent of diphtheria cases also have strep as a secondary infection in the throat.) Diagnosis is made by appropriate cultures of the nose and throat.

Home Treatment

It is imperative that children be routinely immunized for diphtheria during infancy. Three shots are required the first six months of life. Routine boosters are required at 18 to 24 months and at age five. Boosters are further required every ten years thereafter for a lifetime. There is no home treatment for diphtheria, but if your child has not been immunized every cough, sore throat, or case of croup could be the onset of diphtheria.

Precautions

● If your child is not up-to-date on immunization against diphtheria be sure to inform the doctor treating your child. Diphtheria may be the furthest thought from your doctor's mind. ● Consider that an unimmunized child can contract diphtheria from a well child or from an adult who is a carrier.
● Never travel to an underdeveloped country where diphtheria is prevalent without immunization.

Doctor's Treatment

If your doctor suspects diphtheria, he can diagnose and treat the disease. Diphtheria antitoxin, steroids, large doses of penicillin or erythromycin, are effective therapy if started early enough. A tracheostomy may be required if the condition is severe.

Related Topics: Coughs, Croup, Immunizations, Infectious Mononucleosis, Pneumonia, Sore Throat, Strep Throat

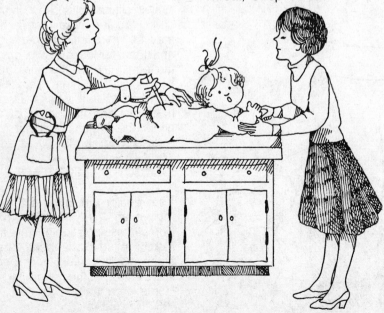

An unimmunized child is in danger of diphtheria with every cough or sore throat.

DISLOCATED ELBOW

Description

A dislocated elbow (Malgaigne's subluxation) is the only common dislocation in young children. Actually, a dislocated elbow is an incomplete dislocation, therefore more properly called a "subluxation." Also known as "nursemaid's elbow," it frequently occurs between one and three years of age and is rare beyond four.

The elbow is composed of two separate joints. The larger is a hinge joint that allows the forearm to bend and to extend in relation to the upper arm. The less obvious joint of the elbow is between the upper ends of the two bones of the forearm (radius and ulna) and allows the forearm to rotate, to turn the palm up and down. It is this radioulnar joint that is partially dislocated when there is a sudden yank on the child's hand or wrist as the parent attempts to save the child from a stumble and fall. It may also be the result of a child being swung around by the wrists in a game or by his grabbing a handhold to prevent falling.

Once the accident occurs, immediate pain results and is located anywhere from the elbow to the wrist. The child refuses to use the affected arm, clutching it to his side with the good arm. Swelling of the wrist and hand develops several hours later.

Diagnosis

If the history is accurate and the child holds his arm with palm facing back, the diagnosis is obvious. Attempts to turn the palm forward cause pain. Without history of a yanked arm, diagnosis is more difficult. The most common incorrect diagnosis is that the child has an injured wrist.

Home Treatment

The first time the condition occurs it is best to have a doctor treat it. A dislocated elbow tends to be recurrent, however, and having observed the treatment once, parents can frequently do it themselves. The corrective maneuver consists of bending the elbow to a 90-degree angle, squeezing the two bones of the forearm together near the elbow with one hand and sharply twisting the wrist so that the palm faces directly upward. **Caution:** Do not attempt this without having the procedure demonstrated. If this maneuver is done within a few hours of the occurrence, a sharp snap or click is heard and actually felt near the elbow. The child is immediately relieved of pain and can use his arm freely.

Precautions

● If history does not fit the classical description do not attempt to reduce the dislocation. A fracture of a forearm bone can produce a similar clinical picture. ● If the elbow is dislocated for more than a few hours, correction may be more difficult because of the swelling, and then for one to two days after correction the arm may still be sore and not fully usable. ● The joint remains susceptible to resubluxation for three to four weeks. Be careful. ● Make a habit of lifting your child by his upper arms or under the armpits and not by pulling on hands, wrists, or forearms.

Doctor's Treatment

Your doctor will confirm the diagnosis and may require an X ray to rule out fracture. Sometimes, positioning the arm for the X ray results in an inadvertent cure. After the diagnosis is certain, your doctor will reduce subluxation in the manner described under Home Treatment.

Related Topic: Fractures

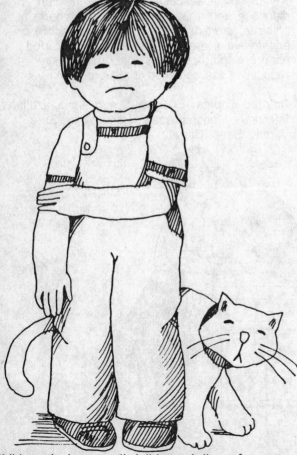

Children who have so-called dislocated elbow often carry the affected arm with the palm facing backward.

Description

Before or after birth, a baby's hip socket on one or both sides may develop too shallowly. Eventually, the thigh bone (femur) dislocates from the socket before or at the time the child stands and walks. The cause is not known, although some cases seem to be inherited, and some are caused by the abnormal position of the legs *in utero*.

If the condition is not diagnosed until dislocation has occurred correction is more difficult. If not corrected before the child walks the child will limp if the dislocation is one-sided and waddle if the dislocation is bilateral.

Diagnosis

If the condition is one-sided parents may notice that one leg is moved more than the other or that the folds of the buttocks or the creases on either side of the groin do not match. A doctor will suspect dislocation by appearance of these signs, by the limited ability of the thighs to be rotated outward, and by a "clunking" sound which is made by the hip when put through a series of movements. Diagnosis must always be confirmed by X rays of both hips.

Home Treatment

Dislocation of the hip(s) is a disabling condition if not treated early and properly. There is no home treatment until the condition is identified by the doctor.

Precautions

● Be sure that your baby is thoroughly examined (while completely undressed) by your doctor at regular, periodic "well-baby" visits. Your doctor should evaluate his hips at each visit until the baby is older than one year. Call any asymmetry of legs to your doctor's attention.

Doctor's Treatment

Your baby should be carefully examined for dislocated hips during each check-up. Your doctor will order X rays if the disorder is suspected. (The diagnosis is not usually made at birth but becomes more obvious with passing months.) As soon as the diagnosis is made you should consult an orthopedic specialist. If the hip is not yet dislocated the doctor will treat with a special pillow positioned to keep the thighs spread or with a body splint or cast. If the hip is already dislocated surgery may be required. Early diagnosis is based upon your alertness and that of your doctor and is the key to easier treatment and perfect, permanent results.

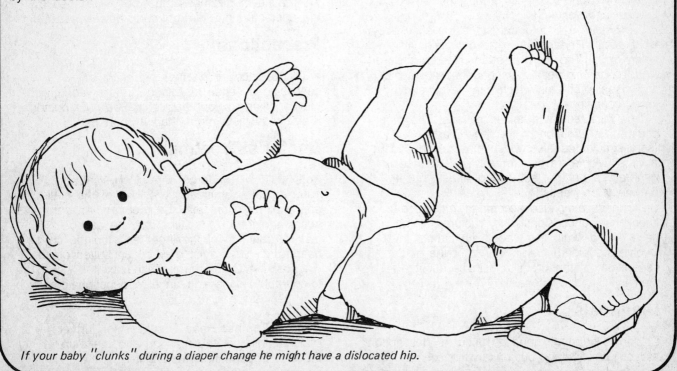

If your baby "clunks" during a diaper change he might have a dislocated hip.

DIZZINESS

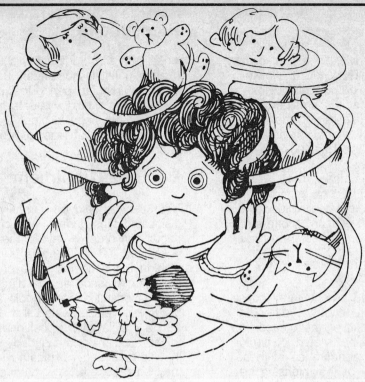

A feeling of dizziness could be caused by any of several conditions; some of them are serious.

Description

Dizziness (vertigo) is the sensation the patient has that he is spinning around or that the environment is turning around the patient. It is a sense of rotation and can be experienced normally by twirling rapidly in one spot until the room reels. Dizziness results in a difficulty in maintaining one's balance and, if prolonged, in nausea and vomiting.

If possible, it is important to establish exactly what a child means when he complains of being dizzy. The word is often used by children to describe faintness, lightheadedness, nausea, and visual problems which can be caused by many conditions.

True dizziness has limited causes. The most common is infection of the inner ear (semi-circular canals), which may be caused by a virus (Meniere's syndrome). This disease is generally a benign, self-curing illness, but it may last for weeks.

Dizziness may also accompany middle ear infections, concussions, and fractures of the base of the skull. It is seen with tumors that involve the eighth cranial nerve or the cerebellum of the brain, and in cases of meningitis and encephalitis.

Diagnosis

Diagnosis depends upon an accurate description by your child, plus your observation of his loss of balance and jerking motions of eyes when directed to one side or the other (nystagmus).

Home Treatment

Dimenhydrinate, available in several over-the-counter preparations, often relieves the sensation of dizziness (consult your pharmacist). The cause of dizziness must be established by the doctor for proper treatment, however.

Precautions

● Try to discover whether the child is describing a sense of rotation before reporting the condition to your doctor. ● See your doctor if dizziness lasts more than a short period.

Doctor's Treatment

Your child will undergo careful physical and neurological examinations. X rays of the skull and a blood count may be required. An ear, nose, and throat specialist may be asked to test the function of the inner ear and the child's hearing. A neurologist may be consulted on the diagnosis. A CAT (computerized axial tomography) scan and an electroencephalogram may be necessary.

Related Topics: Read Deafness for further understanding of the function and make-up of the ear, Encephalitis, Meningitis

Description

The only material that normally comes from the ear canal is wax (cerumen). Ordinarily brown, earwax may be beige or even yellowish if mixed with water from bath, shower, or when swimming. Normally, earwax has only a mild odor, contains no blood, and never flows out in abundance.

Any other material discharging from the ear canal signals a potentially serious condition. It may be a symptom of a middle ear infection; a boil in the ear canal; swimmer's ear; rupture of the eardrum by injury or infection; a foreign body in the ear canal; tumor of the middle ear (cholesteotoma); or fracture of the base of the skull. Abnormal discharge may be thin and watery, bloody, odorous, cheesy, green, yellow, or white.

Diagnosis

Unless it clearly represents typical earwax, any drainage from the ear canal should be considered abnormal and should be promptly seen by a physician.

Home Treatment

Pain accompanying a draining ear may be temporarily treated with aspirin or acetaminophen pain relievers (with or without codeine).

Precautions

● Do not pack cotton into a draining ear. Corking the canal may force the discharge back into the middle ear. ● Do not use a cotton swab or any other instrument to remove material still in the canal. ● Do not attempt to wash out a draining ear as the eardrum may be perforated. ● A draining ear should be seen by a doctor within 12 to 24 hours.

Doctor's Treatment

Your doctor will gently clean your child's ear, inspect it, and make a diagnosis. Treatment, depending on what is found in the ear canal, may require oral antibiotics, medicated ear drops, the removal of a foreign body, an X ray of the child's skull or mastoid bone, or surgery for cholesteatoma (tumor of the middle ear). In the case of a perforated eardrum, antibiotic therapy may be required for a long time, until the eardrum is healed and hearing is restored. Plastic surgery on the eardrum or an adenoidectomy may be necessary.

Related Topics: Deafness, Earaches, Swimmer's Ear

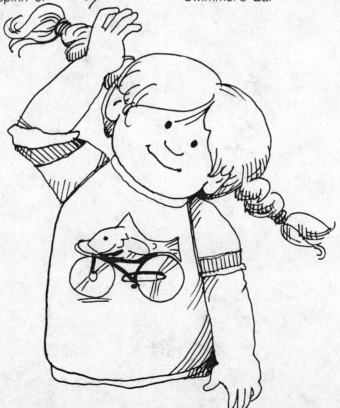

Discharge other than earwax from the ear is abnormal.

DYSENTERY

Description

In popular usage dysentery is taken to mean a severe form of diarrhea. More accurately, it is an infection of the intestinal tract caused by one of several specific bacteria. Dysentery causes diarrhea, but it is a distinct disease.

The causative germs are salmonella and shigella bacteria. Typhoid bacilli are one type of salmonella. Dysentery may also be caused by amebae (amebic dysentery). Some doctors include cholera as a form of dysentery.

Dysentery is the result of eating contaminated food, milk, or water or may be contracted from someone who has the disease or is a carrier of dysentery. The diarrhea is often severe, and is commonly bloody. Prolonged, high fever (103°F to 105°F) and prostration may accompany the disease. Complications include arthritis, meningitis, and perforation of the intestines.

Diagnosis

Any diarrhea should be suspected of being dysentery, especially if it is severe or bloody. Culture of the stools and microscopic examination for amebae and other parasites confirms the diagnosis. Cultures of the blood and urine are sometimes performed as well as tests for the presence of specific antibodies in the blood.

Home Treatment

Treatment at home is the same as for diarrhea but also requires your doctor's decision regarding specific medications.

Precautions

● When traveling, beware of unknown sources of food and water. ● If you suspect dysentery, isolate the patient and dispose of stools carefully. ● Practice good hygiene. ● Report severe or bloody diarrhea to your doctor.

Doctor's Treatment

Your doctor will probably hospitalize your child for treatment and isolation. Specific antibiotics are available. It is mandatory to report diagnosed cases to health authorities.

Related Topics: Arthritis, Diarrhea, Meningitis

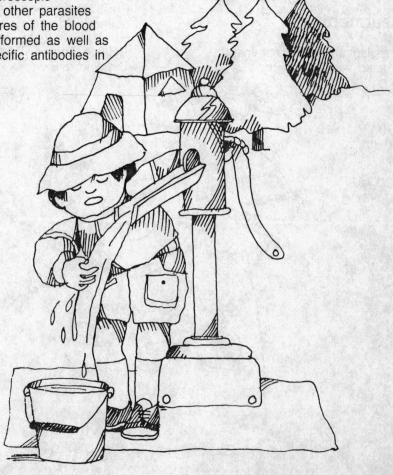

Dysentery can result from drinking contaminated water.

Description

Earaches occur at any age from infancy on, but with decreasing frequency after age eight. Earaches may be: mild or excruciatingly painful; constant or intermittent, or present only with chewing, burping, or nose blowing. They may or may not be accompanied by fever, signs of head cold, or diminished hearing.

The most common cause of an earache is blockage of the eustachian tube (which connects the nose with the middle ear), the result of a nasal allergy, a head cold, infected adenoids, and swimming in fresh or chlorinated water. This blockage causes the formation of a vacuum in the middle ear, pressure changes on the eardrum, and secretion of fluid into the airspace of the middle ear. If obstruction of the eustachian tube persists, infection of the middle ear with pus formation (otitis media) may develop promptly. If the eardrum ruptures, ear discharge develops.

An earache may result from foreign objects in the ear canal or from impacted earwax or from pain in the jaw or molar teeth. Boils may develop in the ear canal from scratching or digging in the ear with bobby pins, hair pins, fingernails, or cotton swabs.

Complications of untreated middle ear infections include mastoiditis, meningitis, and perforated and draining ear. Both middle and outer ear infections can cause swollen, tender lymph nodes.

Diagnosis

If your child is too young to communicate the location of pain, prolonged crying should always be suspected of signifying earache. This is particularly so if the infant has a head cold, congested nose, pulls on his ear, or has recently gone swimming.

The pain of an obstructed eustachian tube is apt to be intermittent, low-grade, and affected by chewing or swallowing. Progression to an abscessed middle ear (otitis media) usually causes intense, often throbbing pain. If the eardrum ruptures, pain quickly abates.

The pain from an infection in the canal, a boil in the canal, a foreign body, or impacted cerumen (earwax) is mild at first and gradually builds. Gentle pressure aggravates pain.

Home Treatment

Any ear pain can be temporarily controlled by aspirin or acetaminophen, plus codeine if necessary. Gentle heat applied to the ear may relieve pain but occasionally worsens it. Anesthetic ear drops must penetrate to the eardrum, and some ear, nose, and throat doctors prefer that they not be used. Nose drops and oral decongestants may open the eustachian tube for an earache accompanied by nasal congestion or allergy.

Precautions

● Children with congested noses should not go swimming. ● Babies under three years should not submerge their heads under water. ● Early treatment of head colds and nasal allergies with nose drops and oral decongestants may prevent some ear problems. ● Children susceptible to swimmer's ear should have their ear canals cleaned by a doctor at the start of each season and preventive ear drops instilled at the end of each swimming day. ● Persistent (more than a few hours) and severe earaches should be seen by your doctor.

Doctor's Treatment

The cause of pain will be established by careful inspection of your child's ears, nose, throat, and neck. For otitis media your doctor will prescribe antibiotics by mouth for five to ten days or until the ear is normal. Nose drops, oral decongestants, and anti-allergy medications also may be prescribed.

Related Topics: Draining Ear, Lymph Nodes—Infection Fighters, Meningitis, Swimmer's Ear

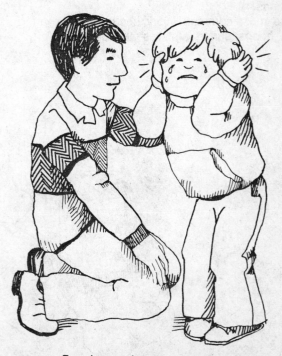

Earaches can be excruciatingly painful.

EARRING PROBLEMS

Description

Pierced ears frequently are the cause of problems involving the earlobes. These are not only annoying in nature but are occasionally serious. Three categories of trouble are infection, eczema (contact dermatitis), and injury. At fault may be the failure of the ear piercer to instruct girls properly.

Infection of the earlobes immediately after operation is caused by lack of proper sterile technique. Infection occurring weeks later is usually from failure to leave "training" (post) earrings in place or to care for them adequately. Infections that occur after the first month are the result of improper insertion of the earrings.

The most frequent errors are inserting earrings whose posts are too short for your child's lobes or pushing the guards too far in along the posts. Both of these mistakes cause injury to the skin of the lobe due to pressure, and infection quickly sets in. Sometimes infection is introduced by using unclean earrings, or by pulling down the lobe to insert the post. This practice curves the straight channel the piercer has made and results in scratching of the lining with the end of the post; the scratches then become infected.

Eczema develops from sensitivity to the metals used as alloys in inexpensive earrings. The skin of the ear lobe becomes red, scaly, itchy, and infected. Signs of infection are swelling, redness, lumps in the lobes, tenderness, discharge, and rawness around the openings.

The most common injury occurs from wearing large hoops during athletics and dancing. An accidental entanglement with the hoop can tear the earlobe neatly in half.

Diagnosis

Any redness, irritation, or scaliness of the skin of the earlobe, and any tenderness, discharge, or lumps are abnormal.

Home Treatment

At the first sign of any abnormality remove the earrings, and leave them out until the condition is corrected. Infection often is impossible to cure with earrings in place. If infection is already well established, the channels may heal closed and require repiercing. Apply antibiotic ointment to the front and back of the lobes. Soak your child's earlobes in a warm Epsom salts solution (a quarter cup to a pint of water). If infected or condition does not respond to therapy or if it is severe, see your doctor.

Precautions

● Ask piercer for detailed instructions. ● Inquire whether piercer will treat complications if they should occur. ● Leave training earrings in for one month, turn them daily, and splash the fronts and backs with alcohol.

Doctor's Treatment

Oral antibiotics may be required to cure infection. If the earlobe is badly lacerated plastic surgery may be necessary. He may prescribe a steroid ointment if eczema is present and infection is not.

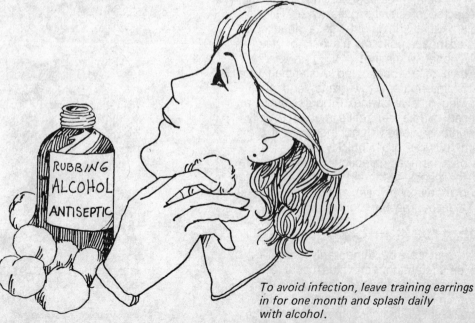

To avoid infection, leave training earrings in for one month and splash daily with alcohol.

Description

Eczema is a common, noncontagious rash in children. Generally, it starts between the neonatal period and age two, but sometimes later. Eczema may disappear after age two or appear off-and-on throughout childhood. Usually it begins on the cheeks ("clown" eczema) and around the mouth and crops up on the buttocks or elsewhere. The characteristic location is behind the knees and in the folds of the elbows. Eczema rarely covers the entire body. It sometimes takes the form of round coin-like patches scattered on the body (nummular eczema).

The eczema rash is dry, slightly scaly, pink, and itchy and becomes red from rubbing and scratching. The skin thickens from rubbing and may bleed. Lesions may become moist and infected from scratching. There is no fever or other symptoms, except in the presence of a secondary infection.

The cause of eczema is questionable but the condition is inherited. Children who have eczema often develop other allergies such as hay fever and asthma later. Eczema sometimes represents an allergic reaction to foods, beverages, and medications (including vitamin supplements). It also may represent a reaction to soaps, detergents, materials (e.g., wool, synthetics, stretch-cotton), dyes, (particularly red and blue), water softeners, cosmetics, metals, and plastics.

Diagnosis

Diagnosis is made by the characteristic appearance of an itchy rash in the locations described. Often it occurs in combination with seborrhea. When in nummular form, eczema may be confused with ringworm and pityriasis rosea.

Home Treatment

Try to treat eczema at home before calling on your doctor's help; home treatment is best except in severe or infected cases. Stop any foods, beverages, and medications started within a month of the rash breaking out. If the rash does not improve in four to seven days in a child under one year stop all foods and beverages most likely to cause eczema: cow's milk (substitute soybean formula) and milk products, wheat flour products, eggs, citrus fruits (including orange juice), chocolate, nuts (and peanut butter), fish and shellfish, tomatoes (tomato juice), and tropical fruits (desserts and drinks). In children over one year stop all the above foods except milk, eggs, and wheat

products. In addition, halt candies, ice cream, spices (not salt), corn, and berries. At any age look for and eliminate possible contactants.

Ointments for eczema for use at home contain coal-tar derivatives and are safe to use, but their use obscures the initial investigation. Use a humidifier to avoid dry air and bathe the child sparingly with mild soaps such as Lowila, Basis, Oilatum, or Aveeno.

If eczema disappears following the above procedure, reintroduce foods one at a time at weekly intervals to detect the offenders. If the condition is not better in one week, see your doctor.

Precautions

• As new foods are added to your infant's diet observe him carefully for any sign of rash. • If your infant is allergic to soy formula as well as milk, your doctor will recommend a nonsoy, nonmilk formula. • Breast-fed infants are rarely allergic to any substance in their mother's diet. • Coal-tar ointments increase sensitivity to sunburn.

Doctor's Treatment

Help your doctor find the cause of eczema by trying a home cure first and noting what doesn't work and what seems to help. Inform your doctor, too, of any similar cases in older siblings. Your doctor may prescribe steroid creams, ointments, or lotions to ease the rash. Oral steroids will not be prescribed unless eczema is severe and then only briefly. Oral antibiotics may be ordered if eczema is infected.

Related Topics: Cradle Cap, Pityriasis Rosea, Ringworn

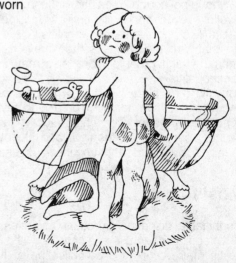

A child with eczema should be bathed sparingly, using mild soap.

ENCEPHALITIS

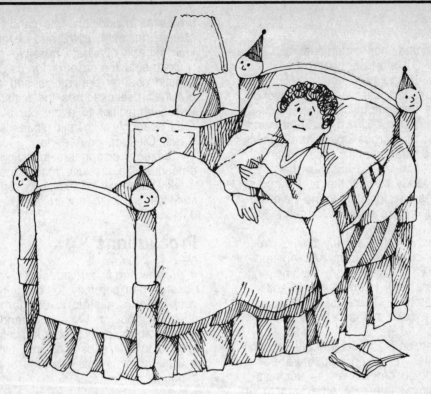

Encephalitis may start with symptoms of the common cold.

Description

Encephalitis is an inflammation of the brain. The causes are innumerable and include poisons, bacteria, vaccines, and parasites. But most cases are caused by viruses, many of which are familiar in relation to such diseases as mumps, measles, rubella, chicken pox, herpes, mononucleosis, hepatitis, and influenza. The whooping cough bacterium can cause encephalitis, as can the vaccines used to prevent whooping cough, measles, influenza, rabies, yellow fever, and typhoid. The vaccines are far less likely to cause encephalitis, however, than are the illnesses they prevent. Lead, mercury, and other poisons also may cause encephalitis.

Encephalitis may start with the symptoms of a common cold. Either no fever or a high fever (105°F) may be present. The child usually has a headache, vomits, is disoriented, and sleepy. Occasionally convulsions and unconsciousness may occur.

Diagnosis

If a recognizable disease is present (measles, mumps, whooping cough) symptoms of encephalitis may occur as a complication of the primary illness. History of exposure to poisons may arouse suspicions.

The most clear-cut physical indication of encephalitis is a stiff neck. A child with the condition will be unable to flex his neck forward to touch his chest with his chin while his mouth is closed. Sometimes the child cannot sit up without supporting himself with both hands braced behind him in tripod fashion. **This is a life-threatening situation.**

Home Treatment

None. See your doctor.

Precautions

● If your child has a severe reaction to any of the vaccines listed above, be sure to tell your doctor before a booster of the vaccine is given.

Doctor's Treatment

Hospitalization may be required. Diagnosis is made on the basis of history; spinal tap; blood count; recovery of organism from spinal fluid, nose, throat, and stools; and upon the presence of antibodies in the patient's blood. There is specific treatment available for only a few types.

Related Topics: Common Cold, Convulsions with Fever, Immunizations, Measles, Mumps, Whooping Cough

Description

Allergic reactions of the eyes (vernal catarrh) may involve the transparent covering (conjunctiva) of the whites of the eyes (sclerae) and the inside of both lids, may involve the skin of the lids and around the eyes or both. They are caused by a wide variety of substances carried to the eyes by the air or hands. Seasonal, airborne materials are tree pollens, grass, ragweed, and other pollens. Nonseasonal materials include animal danders, house dust, feathers, and molds. Those irritants that are carried by the hands are innumerable, but include nail polish, household products, materials from stuffed toys, and finger paints.

The whites of the eyes become red and itchy, the eyes water, but no pus is formed. Occasionally, the whites become visibly swollen with clear gelatinous material (chemosis). The eyelids become swollen and red. The skin of the eyelids may be smooth or rough and scaly. Pouches beneath eyes may become swollen and bluish and resemble shiners. (Other symptoms of allergies include sneezing, a runny and itching nose, coughing, and wheezing.)

Diagnosis

Chemosis is an absolute diagnosis of allergy. Other typical signs are itching without pain and tearing without pus formation. Eye allergies can be proven in your doctor's office by immediate improvement after instillation of one drop of steroid eye drops.

Home Treatment

Oral antihistamines usually help. Eye drops containing phenylephrine or ephedrine bring temporary relief. Cold compresses to eyes may also ease the discomfort. Identifying and, when possible, avoiding the offending substance is clearly the best solution.

Precautions

● If pus or pain is present, the condition is probably not an allergy. ● If the pupil is dilated and slow to respond to light, ● if home treatment is not effective in 24 hours, ● or if vision is affected, see your doctor.

Doctor's Treatment

Your doctor will examine the outside and inside of your child's eyes. Steroid or epinephrine drops are effective but only safe after a doctor's examination. Skin tests may be suggested to help identify the substances causing the irritation. Desensitization shots over an extended period are rarely recommended.

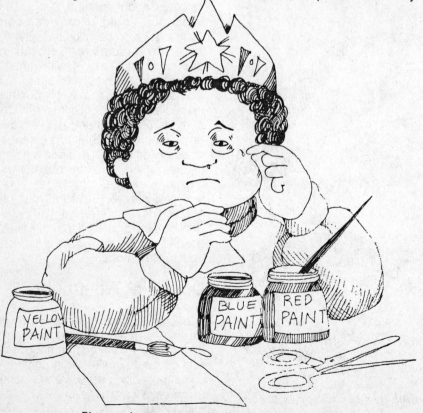

Finger paints can cause an allergic reaction in the eye.

EYE INJURIES

Description

The eyeball is a fragile, hollow sphere not even one-eighth inch thick, within which are many complex and delicate structures. Fortunately, it is well protected by its bony socket and the eyelids.

The eye can be injured by small objects like sand or metallic splinters which land on or become embedded in the surface or which penetrate to the inside of the eye. Sharp objects such as fingernails, knives, and fishhooks can scratch the surface and penetrate the eye. Dull objects such as squash balls and baseball bats can jar the eye and dislodge its internal structures. A tiny speck in the eye may lodge on the surface or hide under the lid.

Diagnosis

When the eyeball is injured, the pain often will cause the victim involuntarily to close his eyelids tightly; light may be painful. The eye must be scrupulously examined to determine the seriousness of the damage. If your child cannot easily open his eye for examination do not attempt to force it open; any damage may be compounded. See your doctor promptly.

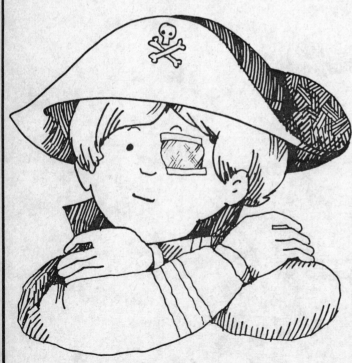

Eye injuries can be very dangerous; be cautious about home treatment.

If your child can open his eye, look carefully for all of the following: free blood coming from the eyeball (do not be misled by blood from a cut near the eye that may have run into the eye); any differences in the pupil of the affected eye compared to the good eye (larger? smaller? different color?); any difference in the color or position of the iris (colored part of the eye); any sign of collapse of the eyeball; puddling of red blood in front of the iris; and blurring of vision. (If present, see below.) If none of these is present you may safely look for foreign objects adherent to the eyeball or lodged under the lid.

Home Treatment

If any of the above signs is present, place a soft bandage over the eye and **see your doctor promptly.** If none of the above signs is present and you see a speck on the eyeball or under the lid (and the child is cooperative) you may try to remove the speck by gentle strokes with a cotton swab. In older children, cup may be used. If the speck does not immediately come off, stop. The object may be embedded. **See a doctor.**

Precautions

● The eyeball is delicate and invaluable. Be cautious about treating eye injuries yourself. ● **If a harmful liquid or powder enters the eye** (acids, alkalis, caustics, gasoline), **immediate action is imperative. Seconds count!** Hold the eye open and flush it with pints of cool water. If available put your child into a cool shower, clothes and all, and wash out his eye. Then, immediately take child to your doctor for further care. ● Do not attempt to remove a fishhook or any other object that has penetrated the eye. ● Some golf balls explode and cause eye injuries if they are unwound. ● **Beware!** Carbon dioxide cartridges and spray cans explode violently in fires. Be sure your child knows this. ● Machine sanders, paint removers, and grindstones throw off particles. Protective glasses and supervision are essential to protect your child's eyes.

Doctor's Treatment

A doctor can easily anesthetize the eye and examine it internally and externally without pain or damage. Your doctor may stain the eyeball with drops to make small injuries and foreign objects readily visible. Areas inside and outside of the eye can be examined with a special microscope.

Description

Tears form in the tear glands that lie within the bony eye sockets above the eyeballs. These glands continuously produce fluid that flows across the eyeballs and down the slender ducts that connect the inner angle of each eye with the nose (nasolacrimal ducts). The two openings into each tear duct are pinpoint in size and can be seen at the innermost edge of the upper and lower lids. If the tear glands fail to produce fluid constantly (an extremely rare condition in children), the eyeballs dry out and, unless the condition is corrected, blindness follows.

In newborns, the openings (puncta) into the tear ducts are often too small and may be further blocked by the silver nitrate or other drops instilled into the eyes at birth to prevent eye infections. This condition may result in tears flowing from the temple side of the baby's eye even when the infant is not crying. Occasionally, instead of normal eye fluid, opaque green or yellow pus will collect in the eye. This discharge will further obstruct the tiny tear ducts.

If the nasolacrimal duct becomes obstructed at the nose end, tearing and possible secondary infection will occur. Obstruction at the nose end can be present at birth or may be caused by a nose cold or allergy. When the nose end is blocked, the nasolacrimal sac between the eye and the side of the nose may swell with fluid and be visible as a distinct lump the size of a green pea.

Diagnosis

Tearing of one or both eyes in infants is so common as to be considered normal; it is harmless. The appearance of pus in the eye, redness and rawness at the outer angle of the eyelids, or swelling with or without redness of the tear sac may require treatment.

Home Treatment

Simple tearing may be ignored. Redness of the skin at the outer angle or the presence of pus may be treated with antibiotic eye drops. If the tear sac is also swollen, gentle milking and massage may be necessary. Your doctor will instruct you.

Precautions

● If home treatment is undertaken, improvement should be obvious within 24 hours. If there is no improvement, notify your doctor. ● If improvement is prompt, continue treatment until the eye is clear for at least two days.
● Recurrence is common; save the eye drops for possible future use.

Doctor's Treatment

Your doctor's treatment is the same as home treatment. Your doctor can demonstrate the proper method of massaging the tear sac if needed. If the condition persists past one year of age, your doctor may refer your child to an ophthalmologist who may dilate the nasolacrimal duct under general anesthesia.

Related Topic: Conjunctivitis

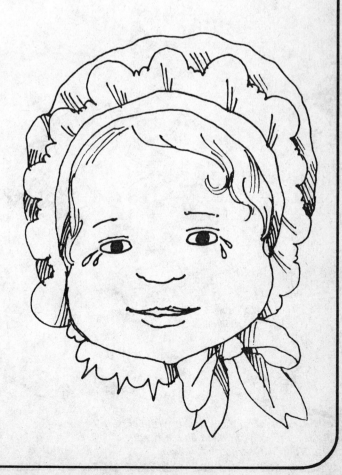

Infants commonly tear in one or both eyes; redness or swelling, however, is cause for concern.

FAINTING

Description

Fainting is a temporary loss of consciousness caused by the involuntary (autonomic) nervous system. It can be initiated by pain, physical fatigue, low blood sugar, a disturbing scene, sudden fright, and other strong emotions. The child experiences light-headedness, narrowing of visual fields, clamminess, and sometimes mild nausea just before unconsciousness. An observer may notice a paleness or "green color" and a glazed look in the eyes at the onset of a faint. Occasionally there will be mild, convulsive movements while the child is unconscious. Rarely will control of the urine or stools be lost. Consciousness will be recovered within a few minutes and the child will probably not remember the event.

Fainting is common in pre-adolescent and adolescent children. It often occurs after the child has gone without eating for an extended period of time. A partial faint (lightheadedness and dizziness) or a complete faint is also common when a teenager abruptly changes position, for example jumping up from a reclining or sitting position. It also can occur in a dentist's chair caused by a combination of pain, anxiety, and turning the head sharply to one side (from pressure of the collar against the carotid body—found within the walls of the carotid artery in the neck).

Diagnosis

Diagnosis is made by consideration of the circumstances, plus a complete, rapid recovery (which suggests it's nothing more serious than an isolated spell). The pulse at the wrist may be diagnostically feeble and slow or not present at all. The heart beat (ear against chest) is slow, usually 50 beats per minute or slower.

Home Treatment

The only danger in fainting is the injury your child may incur from a fall. Try to catch him as he goes down, and lay him flat on his back, elevating his legs to return the blood to the head. Although not mandatory, the coolness from an open window or air conditioner may help. Keep your child down for five to ten minutes after consciousness returns.

An alternative treatment if your child is not yet unconscious, is to have him sit with his head between his knees. Place your hand on the back of his head and have him strain to sit up while you hold his head down. This maneuver forces extra blood into the head.

If she feels faint, have her sit with her head between her knees. Place your hand on her head and have her strain to sit up while you push down.

Precautions

● Sometimes a first convulsion is mistaken for fainting. If fainting is recurrent or if other signs of epilepsy are present see your doctor. ● If blueness of skin (cyanosis) is observed during an apparent faint or if your child is not completely well before and after fainting, consult your doctor. Extremely rare heart conditions might simulate fainting. ● If you use smelling salts to revive your child (certainly not necessary), be careful not to burn the membranes of the nose.

Doctor's Treatment

Your doctor will treat fainting the same as you would at home. Although fainting cannot be diagnosed after the faint is over, various causes of unconsciousness can be ruled out. Your doctor may require an electrocardiogram, electroencephalogram, blood chemistries, or chest X ray.

Related Topics: Convulsions without Fever, Dizziness

Description

Erythema infectiosum, or fifth disease, is a moderately contagious, childhood disease caused by a virus that has not yet been identified. The incubation period averages two weeks but may range from one to four weeks. Usually the patient has little or no fever and feels minimally or not at all ill. The disease is characterized by the sudden appearance of a bright red rash on the cheeks, making it appear as though the child has been slapped. Then a pink rash like a lace tablecloth (reticulated) appears on the trunk and extremities. The condition can last two to forty days and may itch. In older children and young adults, symptoms of headache, sore throat, runny nose, loss of appetite, and nausea may occur.

Diagnosis

Contraction of fifth disease usually is obvious from the appearance of the typical rash, especially if an epidemic is current in the neighborhood or school. It is occasionally confused with rubella, rashes from medications, and other viral rashes. The condition is rarely confused with scarlet fever. There are no diagnostic laboratory tests.

Home Treatment

No isolation is required. Public health authorities have deemed it permissible for the child to attend school if fever is absent and the child can tolerate it. Itching can be treated with antihistamines or hydroxyzine.

Precautions

None.

Doctor's Treatment

There is no work for the doctor beyond confirmation of diagnosis.

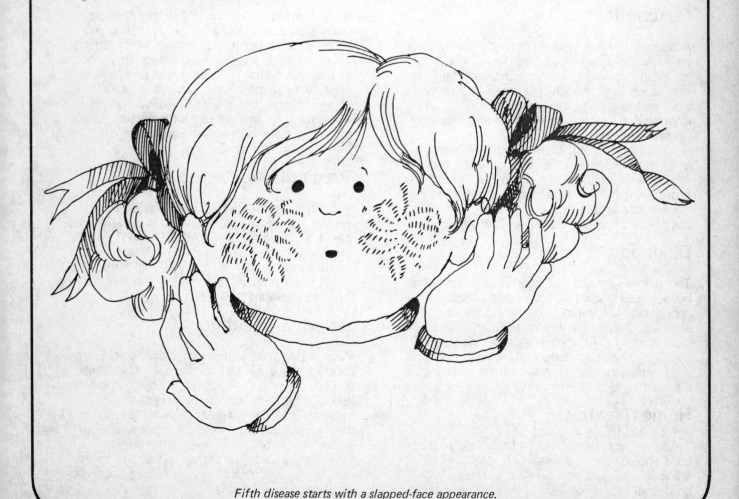

Fifth disease starts with a slapped-face appearance.

FLAT FEET

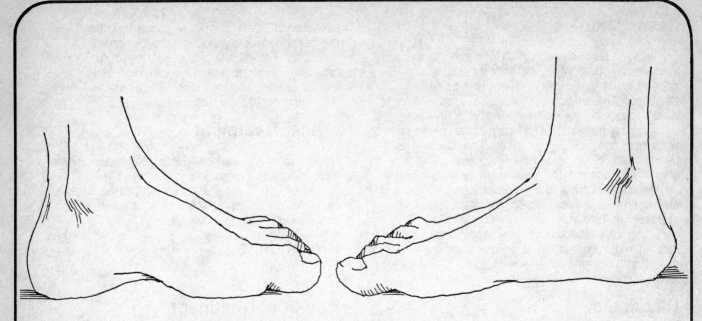

A truly flat-footed child has no arch at all.

Description

A normal, newborn baby does not have arches on its feet. Arches don't start to develop until the child begins to walk unaided, and they do not appear until the child is three to four years old—formed by the developing strength of the leg muscles exerted on the normal bones and ligaments of the feet.

With true flat feet, there is no arch when a child stands; he walks on the inner edge of the foot. This practice breaks down the tops of the shoes from the inside and wears down the inner edges of the heels and soles. The child complains of painful feet after brief exercise.

Diagnosis

The normal condition of your child's feet before he develops arches is sometimes called "physiological flat feet." The presence or absence of an arch at any age can best be judged when your child stands on the tips of his toes. After age three or four years, your child should no longer wear out his shoes in the manner described above.

Home Treatment

To encourage development of the foot your child should not wear walking shoes until he starts to walk unaided on hard surfaces. If a child under three or four years of age breaks down the upper portion of his shoes or wears out the inner edges of the heels before the shoes are outgrown, buy shoes with a stronger counter (the inner part of the back third section. of the upper shoe). If your child past age three appears flat-footed have him tiptoe barefoot five to ten minutes per day. A child over six to eight years of age should walk barefooted on the outer edge of his foot with his toes clenched for ten minutes daily.

Precautions

● Do not use orthopedic shoes or devices without competent professional advice. Thomas heels, scaphoid pads ("cookies"), and orthopedic shoes are expensive if not needed, and they actually may harm normal feet. ● Painful feet after excessive use and exercise do not indicate abnormal feet.

Doctor's Treatment

Your doctor will examine your child's feet carefully while he stands and sits, stands on tiptoes, and walks. Tests for mobility of the joints of the feet, the strength of the foot muscles, and the adequacy of the tendons will be conducted. Your doctor will examine worn shoes and may x-ray your child's feet. Considering all these factors in relation to the child's age, the doctor may prescribe exercises or orthopedic shoes.

FOOD POISONING

Description

The classical form of food poisoning is caused by staphylococci, the same germs that cause boils and impetigo. The germs are introduced into the food during its preparation, and if the food is not properly refrigerated, the germs multiply hourly contaminating the food with a secreted toxin. The foods in which staph germs have the opportunity to grow best are pastries and other starchy foods ordinarily served cold; salads; cold chicken; ham and beef in gelatin; whipped cream; and custards. The staph and their toxins are odorless and tasteless.

Eating contaminated food causes vomiting, abdominal cramps, and diarrhea within one to six hours. Fever may or may not be present. Symptoms last 12 to 24 hours.

A variety of germs other than staph also can cause food poisoning of a milder nature. Two other conditions that are sometimes classified as food poisoning are botulism and dysentery.

Diagnosis

Any vomiting and diarrhea *might* be food poisoning. Diagnosis is usually considered when a number of people who have eaten the same food become ill within hours of one another. Picnics, parties, and eating out in a cafeteria or restaurant where any of the above foods have been prepared in advance and improperly stored may give rise to food poisoning.

Home Treatment

Home treatment is the same as for vomiting and diarrhea.

Precautions

● Do not prepare food that requires refrigeration for your child's lunchbox or a picnic if refrigeration is not available.

Doctor's Treatment

In severe cases hospitalization for administration of intravenous fluids may be required. Local departments of health can investigate outbreaks and trace the source of food poisoning by culturing suspected foods.

Related Topics: Botulism, Diarrhea, Dysentery, Vomiting

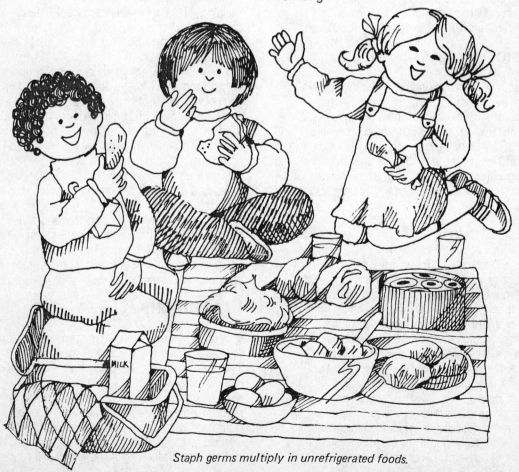

Staph germs multiply in unrefrigerated foods.

FRACTURES

Description

A fracture, a broken bone, and a fractured bone are all the same. Children's bones are still growing, which gives their fractures characteristics that differ from adult fractures. Any deformity caused by a fracture that heals in a poor position tends to be corrected through growth (except if the poor position is one that shortens or rotates the bone). Fractures through the growing cartilage near both ends of long bones may stop growth and cause major deformities. Broken bones heal in less time for children than for adults. All of these traits are even more marked for the very young child.

A fracture may be: *undisplaced* (fragments in normal relationship to each other); *angulated* (fragments form an angle); *displaced* (fragments not aligned); *greenstick* (bone bent but not fractured completely through); *simple* (no break in overlying skin); *compound* (break in overlying skin, introducing possibility of infection); *comminuted* (bone broken into several pieces); *impacted* (broken ends jammed into each other so that fracture site is stable); *chip* (tiny piece of bone knocked off); *spiral* (fracture line corkscrews); *transverse* (fracture line at right angles to long axis of bone); or *oblique* (fracture line at sharp angle to long bone).

Diagnosis

Deformity of the bone is visible or can be felt. Pain is aggravated by attempts to move the broken part, and there is a tenderness to pressure which is most severe at the point of the fracture. The function of the fractured part is limited, and there is swelling at the fracture site. Bruising often develops, but sometimes not until days later and in areas many inches from the fracture.

Home Treatment

Protect the injured part. If the arm or shoulder is fractured, the child will usually immobilize the part in the most comfortable position with his other arm. If a leg or spine fracture is suspected, prevent your child from putting weight on the fracture. If splinting is required for your child's arm or leg a folded pillow is often the best splint. Immobilize the fractured area in a comfortable position and take the child to your doctor.

Obvious fractures usually raise no question of home treatment. Problems arise from borderline cases, as in the following fractures:

Collar bone (clavicle). This is the most common fracture in young children. It occurs from a fall onto the point of the shoulder. There is pain on raising the arm overhead. The entire bone is just beneath the skin so it can be touched carefully with the fingers to feel the point of tenderness, lump, and change in contour compared to opposite clavicle.

Wrist. (lower radius or ulna) This is the most common fracture in older children. It occurs from a fall on an outstretched arm. Unlike a sprain, the most tender point is usually one half inch to two inches above the wrist joint. Also unlike a sprain, it hurts the child to turn the palm up and down.

Elbow (lower humerus). Moderate to marked swelling is present and the most tender point is above or at the joint and also along the inside or outside edge of the bone. Any motion of the forearm causes pain.

Ankle (lower femur or fibula). Unless the break is severe, an ankle fracture is hard to tell from a sprain. The tender point is above the lower tip of the bone rather than at or below the tip.

Foot (metatarsal bones). Five slender bones that make up the instep are often fractured, sometimes just by marching (march fracture) or running. This type of fracture is extremely difficult to diagnose, and even X rays may be normal until one to two weeks after the fracture occurs.

Toes. Unless there is a great deformity or a compound fracture, diagnosis doesn't matter. Put a wad of cotton between the injured toe and those on either side of it, and bind them together with adhesive tape. The fracture will heal perfectly in two to three weeks.

Fingers. If the fracture occurs in the bone beneath the fingernail as might be caused by a slammed door or a hammer blow, it will heal perfectly without treatment unless it is a compound fracture. Other finger fractures are serious if the fractured finger is not straight or if the fracture is compound. Otherwise, splinting for three to four weeks is sufficient. If you suspect fracture take your child to your doctor.

Precautions

● A dangerous, often overlooked fracture is that of the navicular (scaphoid) bone of the wrist. The navicular bone resembles a small cashew nut, is one of eight small bones in the wrist, and lies near the base of the thumb's metacarpal bone. This fracture causes only moderate pain and little swelling, but if it is not treated part of the bone dies, resulting in a permanent deformity. Any point of tenderness in this area after injury should be seen by a doctor. ● Do not move an injured extremity to conform to a splint. Splint a possible fracture in the position found with a wood lath or a pillow (see Home Treatment). ● Do not move your child if there is any possibility of a neck or spine injury.

Doctor's Treatment

Your doctor's treatment will depend largely upon what the X rays show. Open or closed reduction of fracture will be performed with casting or mechanical pinning if necessary.

Related Topics: Dislocated Elbow, Sprains & Dislocations

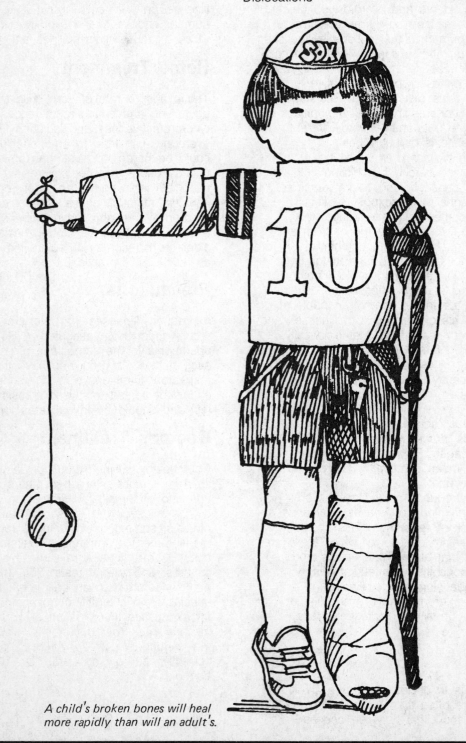

A child's broken bones will heal more rapidly than will an adult's.

FREQUENT ILLNESSES

Description

Parents frequently become concerned that their children are ill too often. Sometimes they are right and corrective action is called for. But frequency of illness is a comparative thing, depending on the number of children in a family and the number of diseases each child is exposed to.

Excluding accidents and allergies, 95 percent of illnesses are caused by germs that live exclusively in humans. Most children's illnesses are caught from other children. Whether a child will catch a disease depends on two things: whether he is exposed to the causative germ and how strong his resistance is. Resistance depends upon general and local immunity.

If your child is frequently ill with different and minor illnesses he is probably being overexposed to sick children or adults. Tonsillitis, followed quickly by chicken pox, viral gastroenteritis, impetigo, and a viral respiratory infection are signs of overexposure. This overexposure comes from attendance at a nursery school that is poorly run or from any mass baby-sitting facility. The number of children in a household also is a factor. In a family of four children each child will have several times as many sicknesses as an only child. Each of the four children is capable of bringing home his or her share of illnesses and shares them with the others. Mathematically, a normal, four-child family could have 16 times as many childhood illnesses as a one-child family.

A child frequently ill with the same illness often has a defect of local resistance. Repeated pneumonia in the same part of a lung suggests a foreign body or abnormality in that area. Recurrent sinus infections imply a malfunction of the nasal passages. Frequent middle ear problems may mean something is wrong with the eustachian tube.

A child with frequent major illnesses or complications of minor sicknesses may have a generalized lack of resistance. This occurs with immune mechanism defects, of which there are several. Colds that always end up as croup, bronchiolitis, bronchitis, or pneumonia may indicate an underlying allergy. Recurrent pneumonia in different parts of the lungs or throughout the lungs may represent cystic fibrosis.

Diagnosis

The first step is to decide whether a child is actually ill more often than his or her peers. Some reports show that between one and twelve years of age the average, normal child will have eight illnesses per year. Other figures show that a first child will seldom be ill during the first year, then have increasingly frequent sicknesses as he or she plays with other children and attends nursery school, kindergarten, and grade school. An infant with siblings will be sick the first year as often as the siblings are. To diagnose too-frequent illnesses in your child you must compare the number and seriousness of the illnesses with those of your child's siblings and peers.

Home Treatment

The exposure rate of your child to illnesses is up to you and your circumstances. Overprotectiveness and isolation from peers, if overdone, can lead to emotional problems which could be harder to treat than physical ones. Overexposure to other children who may be ill, especially at a young age, can lead to almost constant minor illnesses. Keep older children—yours and the neighbor's—from treating your baby as though he is a doll. If an older child becomes ill isolate him from siblings as much as is practical.

Precautions

• Frequent illnesses that interfere with normal growth must be investigated. • Recurrent pneumonia in the same lobe of a lung must be evaluated. • Children who have frequent respiratory infections with a prolonged cough should be tested for cystic fibrosis by a sweat test and should be investigated for allergies.

Doctor's Treatment

Your doctor will help you decide whether your child is ill more often than others of the same age and under similar circumstances. If so your doctor will seek the cause by issuing a barrage of tests, sometimes including a sweat test, measurement of immune globulins, blood count, chest X ray, sinus X rays, nose and throat cultures, and allergy tests. You and your child may be referred to an ear, nose, and throat specialist, an allergist, or to a medical center for exhaustive investigation of all immune mechanisms. Your doctor may also recommend trial of long-term (prophylactic) antibiotics or corrective surgery on ears, nose, or tonsils and adenoids.

Related Topic: Cystic Fibrosis

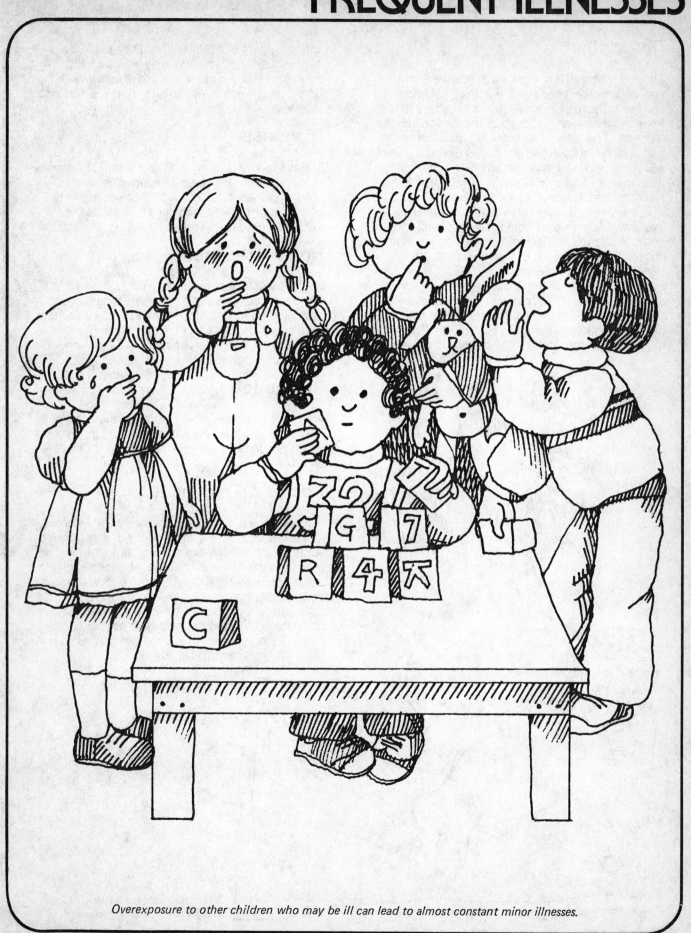

Overexposure to other children who may be ill can lead to almost constant minor illnesses.

FUNNEL CHEST

Description

The breastbone (sternum) is joined to the front end of the ribs which are made of cartilage in children. The diaphragm muscle attaches in front to the lower ribs and to the bottom of the sternum. The ribs of a baby are delicate, and the diaphragm is relatively strong. When some babies breathe in, the diaphragm normally pulls the lower half of the sternum toward the spine, causing a hollow in the center of the chest. This hollow is exaggerated when the flow of air into the lungs is obstructed, as with a stuffed nose, bronchitis, bronchiolitis, pneumonia, and choking; this condition is called *retracting,* a sign of breathing difficulty.

If the sternum is depressed even while the child is at rest and breathing out, a funnel chest exists. If mild or moderate it will cause no harm and will gradually correct itself over the years as the child's ribs become heavier and stronger. But if the condition is severe it may not self-correct and may interfere with breathing and restrict the child's activities. Rarely is it severe enough to displace the heart or threaten its functioning.

Diagnosis

Diagnosis is made by observing the chest of a well child. Severity is estimated when the child breathes out. In marked cases severity and effect on heart and lungs is judged by X ray and fluoroscopy results.

Home Treatment

Retractions of the lower sternum which have not been previously present are an important sign of breathing difficulty in a child. Treatment is directed toward the disease causing the condition. A fixed deformity (true funnel chest) cannot be altered by home treatment.

Precautions

● Don't be alarmed by persistent mild to moderate depression of the sternum in an infant or young child. ● Do not restrict your child's activities.

Doctor's Treatment

If funnel chest is severe and persists without gradual improvement the condition may require surgery. Indications for surgery are cosmetic or signs of limited heart or lung function. Your doctor may order X rays, an electrocardiogram, and measurements of the lung capacity. If the condition is aggravated by chronic nasal obstruction, caused by enlarged adenoids, the adenoids may need to be removed. Your doctor also will treat any nasal allergy.

Related Topic: Breathing Difficulty

A mild or moderate case of funnel chest will gradually correct itself.

GASTROENTERITIS, ACUTE

Description

Acute gastroenteritis is a highly contagious infection of the digestive tract probably caused by viruses, only a few of which have been identified. There is evidence indicating that the disease may also be caused by some types of Escherichia coli bacilli, a normal inhabitant of the human intestines and most of whose members are known to be harmless and even beneficial.

Acute gastroenteritis causes a sudden onset of vomiting or diarrhea and cramps. The disease lasts one to three days, sometimes a week. Fever may be high (104°F), low (101°F). or absent. Blood in diarrhea is rare. Occasionally, there are small amounts of blood in vomitus and petechiae (red spots) of the face if vomiting is severe. The disease is readily transmitted from person to person. The incubation period is one to four days. The disease is not generally serious except in young babies, who may become dehydrated. One attack confers variable, brief, or no immunity against subsequent attacks. Acute gastroenteritis has no relationship to true flu, a disease of the respiratory tract.

Diagnosis

Acute gastroenteritis is usually obvious if there are other cases in the family or neighborhood. It occasionally must be distinguished from dysentery and food poisoning.

Home Treatment

Treat vomiting and diarrhea. Limit food intake to clear liquids until the illness subsides. Acetaminophen is better for relief of fever than aspirin because of a slight tendency of aspirin to aggravate vomiting in some children.

Precautions

● If present in siblings isolate a baby in a room with a closed door. ● Practice good hygiene. Be sure to wash your hands before going from the patient to a baby. ● If a young child develops the disease watch carefully for signs of dehydration.

Doctor's Treatment

Your doctor will confirm the diagnosis by knowledge of what illnesses are current in the community, by history, and by absence of other physical findings on examination. Blood count and a stool culture might be required if diagnosis is in doubt. Otherwise, your doctor's treatment will be the same as home treatment. If there is evidence of dehydration in an infant hospitalization may be necessary in order to administer intravenous fluids.

Related Topics: Appendicitis, Dehydration, Diarrhea/Children, Diarrhea/Infants, Dysentery, Food Poisoning, Vomiting.

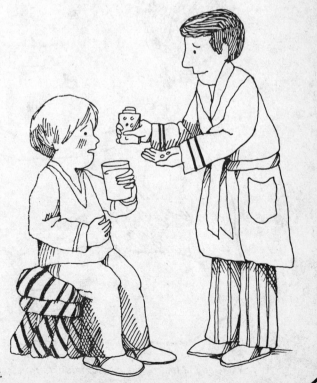

It will pass, but while he has it, offer ailment aids.

GEOGRAPHIC TONGUE

Description

Geographic tongue is a common, harmless patterning of the tongue seen in five to ten percent of infants and children. The cause is unknown. There are no symptoms or discomfort of any sort. One or more smooth, bright red patches appear on the surface of the tongue, and in the course of several days, these patches change size, shape, and location. The general impression is that of a slowly changing map, hence the name. The condition lasts for months to years, and may recur after disappearing.

The usual velvety-and-rough, whitish-pink surface of the tongue is composed of closely packed papillae (taste buds). The smooth, red areas of changing contour on a geographic tongue are made up of papillae that have shrunk or temporarily disappeared (atrophied). Yet there are no discernible changes in the sense of taste, and there is no pain.

Diagnosis

Diagnosis is made on close inspection and from the characteristic appearance of the tongue. No other disease resembles geographic tongue.

Home Treatment

Treating geographic tongue is like treating red hair or blue eyes. No home treatment is required or effective.

Precautions

• Geographic tongue does not indicate a vitamin deficiency, reaction to toothpaste, or any other pathology. • Do not try any home treatment. • Do not instill any concern into your child regarding his geographic tongue.

Doctor's Treatment

Your doctor will reassure you and your child that geographic tongue is not a cause for concern.

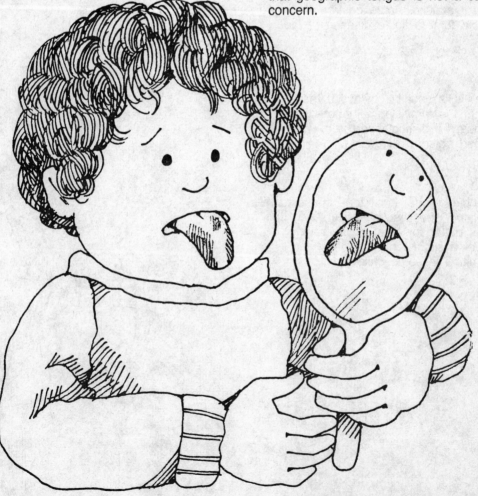

Geographic tongue is a common, harmless patterning of the tongue; it has no other symptoms.

Description

The lymph "glands" of the entire body or of a localized area may become involved in a disease process. When these nodes swell and become mildly tender they are performing their beneficial function of providing antibodies and limiting the spread of germs or other harmful agents. When they continue to swell, become painful and more tender, and redden the overlying skin, they may have been overwhelmed to become part of the disease process.

Generalized enlargement of lymph nodes is part of infectious mononucleosis. Occasionally, swollen glands indicate leukemia, or another malignancy of the blood cells. Chicken pox, being generalized, causes swollen nodes in many areas as might widespread impetigo, boils, or scabies. Rubella causes lymphadenitis at the nape of the neck, behind the ears, and immediately in front of the ears.

When nodes are swollen in one area, a cause exists in that particular area. The cause might be an insect bite, cat scratch, boil, infected wound (even trivial), impetigo, or other infection. If the glands at the back of scalp and behind the ears are swollen look at the scalp on the same side for a cause. If the glands on both sides of the neck are swollen look for cold or infection of upper respiratory tract (sinuses, tonsils, throat). If the glands under the chin are swollen, check for acne of the face, a tooth infection, and canker sores. If the lymph glands in the armpits are swollen evaluate the side of the chest or arm. If the glands of the elbows are swollen check the forearm, hand, and fingers. If the glands of the groin are swollen check the lower abdomen, leg, foot, genitalia, and anal areas.

Diagnosis

Diagnosis depends upon finding the disease that initiated swelling of the glands and then deciding whether the glands themselves require treatment beyond therapy indicated for the primary cause.

Home Treatment

Swollen glands usually require only treatment for the primary problem.

Precautions

● Swollen glands in the neck (and sometimes other locations) of a baby usually require a doctor's treatment because of the infants' limited immunity. ● Any node that continues to increase in size and tenderness or becomes reddened needs a doctor's attention. ● Normal children have visible nodes the size of fresh peas or smaller on sides of neck. These may become prominent when the child turns his head; they are normal.

Doctor's Treatment

Your doctor will seek the cause of swollen glands by conducting a complete examination, including all sites of glands, spleen, and liver. A blood count, heterophile test, chest and kidney X rays, bone marrow examination, and sedimentation rate may be required. Your doctor may treat this condition with antibiotics. The affected gland may be incised and drained or removed as treatment or for a biopsy (culture and microscopic examination).

Related Topics: Boils, Chicken Pox, Impetigo, Infectious Mononucleosis, Leukemia, Lymph Nodes—Infection Fighters, Rubella, Scabies

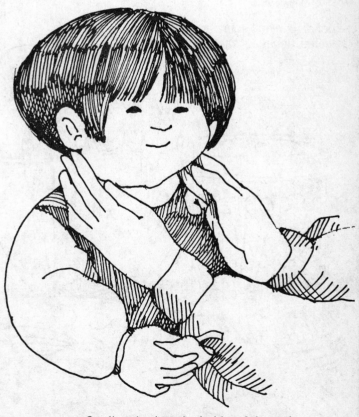

Swollen glands on both sides of the neck can indicate a cold or an infection of the upper respiratory tract.

GOITER

Description

A goiter is a swelling in the neck caused by the enlargement of the thyroid gland. The thyroid gland lies just below and to either side of the larynx (Adam's apple). A normal thyroid is barely (if at all) visible or able to be felt.

A goiter may be present in a newborn infant, especially if the mother is on certain medications, including iodides in antiasthma or cough medicines. Insufficient iodine in your child's diet also can cause a goiter. Once prevalent, this disease is now rare because of general use of iodized table salt and more widespread consumption of seafood (seafood is naturally high in iodine content).

A goiter is most common between ages six and sixteen years and occurs in girls nine times as often as it does in boys. It is most often due to an autoimmune (self-destructive) disease—Hashimoto's thyroiditis—of unknown cause. Enlargement of the thyroid is rarely the result of a malignancy. A goiter may be hyperactive or hypoactive but usually is neither. (See Thyroid.) Generally there are no other symptoms.

Diagnosis

A goiter can be seen and felt. It is often detected because shirt collars or neck jewelry no longer fit. The cause cannot be diagnosed without laboratory tests.

Home Treatment

No home treatment should be attempted until the cause is diagnosed by your doctor.

Precautions

● Do not take medications, even over-the-counter drugs, during pregnancy without your doctor's approval. ● Not all thyroid glands are in the expected anatomical position. Any enlarging lump in the midline of the neck may be a goiter of a misplaced thyroid. A lump should never be removed from this area without first testing to confirm it is not the thyroid gland.

Doctor's Treatment

Complex blood tests, often requiring sophisticated laboratory work, are used to find the cause of a goiter. The treatment for a goiter usually is the administration of oral thyroxine or desiccated thyroid for months or years. Surgery is rarely necessary except for malignancy or when breathing is obstructed in infants.

Related Topic: Thyroid

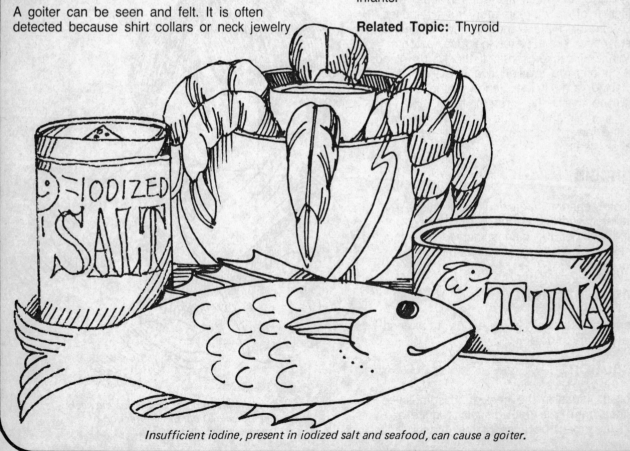

Insufficient iodine, present in iodized salt and seafood, can cause a goiter.

Description

In pre-antibiotic days conjunctivitis in newborns whose mothers had gonorrhea was common. Antibiotics and the compulsory Credé treatment (the administration of silver nitrate solution into the eyes of all newborns) have almost eradicated this previously prevalent cause of blindness.

Today, venereal (sexually transmitted) gonorrhea in adolescent and younger boys and girls is being seen with increasing and alarming frequency. Gonorrhea of the genitalia of boys causes burning on urination and a discharge from the penis. In girls gonorrhea may cause vaginal discharge and abdominal pain, but frequently there are no symptoms at all. A "new" disease being seen in children and caused by gonococcus bacterium is a sore throat and anal infection, with or without fever. (Ordinary throat cultures done for sore throats do not grow the gonococcus, which leads to the erroneous conclusion that the infection is viral and that no antibiotic need be prescribed.)

Diagnosis

Diagnosis is made only by alertness, awareness, and by special culture techniques and microscopic examination of vaginal and penile discharges. Many advocate the practice of taking periodic vaginal cultures at the time of routine school and annual examinations of sexually active girls. Serious consequences, including sterility, may result from untreated cases in females. Most causes are diagnosed by tracing the sexual contacts of the individuals with known cases of gonorrhea.

Home Treatment

None.

Precautions

● Be aware that the disease still exists and that it exists in children of all ages. ● Provide sex education for your children.

Doctor's Treatment

Your doctor will establish the diagnosis by smear and special culture techniques. Although penicillin-resistant gonoccoci are now reported, other new antibiotics are reliably effective. Cases are reportable by law to health departments. Treatment of minors is confidential; parental consent is not required.

Related Topic: Vaginal Discharge

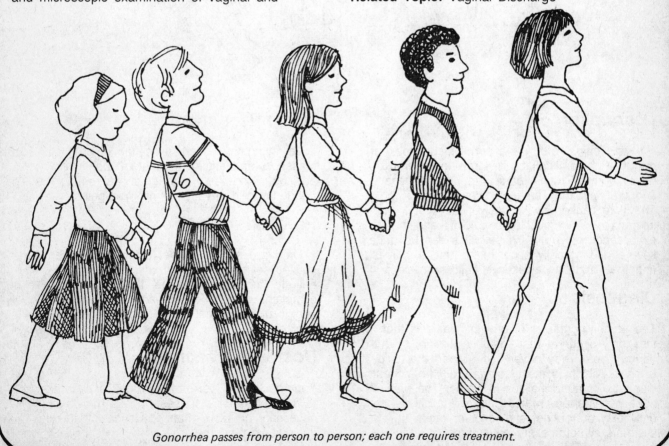

Gonorrhea passes from person to person; each one requires treatment.

GROWING PAINS

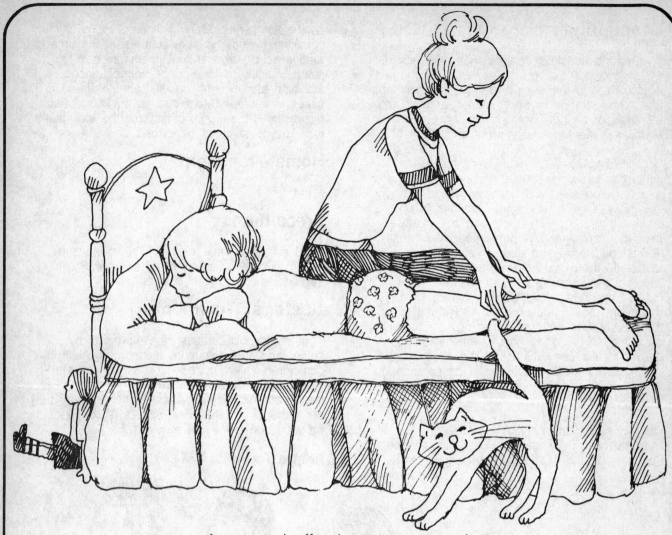

A massage on the affected area can ease sore muscles.

Description

Growing pains refers to a popular concept that is half truth and half myth. Growing children do have "normal" pains, particularly in their legs and feet, but they are not caused by growing. They are caused by excessive use of the immature young muscles and joints and the exuberance of youth. These pains can be quite severe and typically occur in the thighs, calves, and feet, and can awaken a child from sleep.

Diagnosis

The identifying factor of growing pains is that they only occur at rest—usually at night or during naps. They never occur when the child is active which is the time that pain from most diseases or abnormalities is worse. The pain does not interfere with or interrupt a child's daily play or routine, and fever or other systemic symptoms are never present.

Home Treatment

Love, sympathy, local application of heat, massage, and aspirin or acetaminophen are advised. Sometimes sturdier shoes reduce the frequency and severity of growing pains.

Precautions

● One rare bone disease, osteoid osteoma, causes severe bone pain which is almost entirely limited to nighttime. If your child complains of pain in the same spot, frequently, and at night the cause must be checked by your doctor.

Doctor's Treatment

Your doctor will perform a careful examination to rule out other diseases. X rays may be necessary on more than one occasion to rule out osteoid osteoma.

Description

A gum boil is an *apical abscess* that "points" (breaks through the surface) where the lip meets the gum at the site of a decayed tooth. The condition almost always occurs only with a baby tooth, rarely with a permanent one. It is caused by infection reaching the root canal and traveling to the apex of the tooth's root. It is sometimes painful, and the tooth may be tender. Fever is rare. Gum boils are common after a cavity in a tooth has been repaired and filled, and in untreated decayed or injured teeth. The condition appears as a tender pimple which eventually discharges yellow pus.

Diagnosis

Gum boils' typical appearance determines their diagnosis. A gum boil can only be confused with a canker sore, which is ulcerated (dug out), not protruding like a gum boil. Usually the associated tooth is obviously injured (fractured or discolored) or has an untreated or recently filled cavity. The tooth may be tender to tapping or may be slightly loose.

Home Treatment

Give aspirin or acetaminophen for pain. Warm soaks or warm salt water rinses (one-half teaspoonful table salt in one-half glass warm water) will help solve the problem. If a tooth is soon to be lost naturally, the condition can be ignored. The loss of the tooth will provide drainage and the cure.

Precautions

● Premature loss of first- or second-year molars (or permanent six-year molars) can cause later orthodontic calamities. ● Some dentists feel that a gum boil of a deciduous (baby) tooth endangers the unerupted permanent tooth.

Doctor's Treatment

No treatment by your doctor is necessary unless your dentist is unavailable. Your dentist will decide whether to ignore the tooth, pull it, pull it and replace it with a space retainer, or salvage the tooth by performing root-canal work (endodontistry). Antibiotic therapy or incision and drainage through the gum is rarely required.

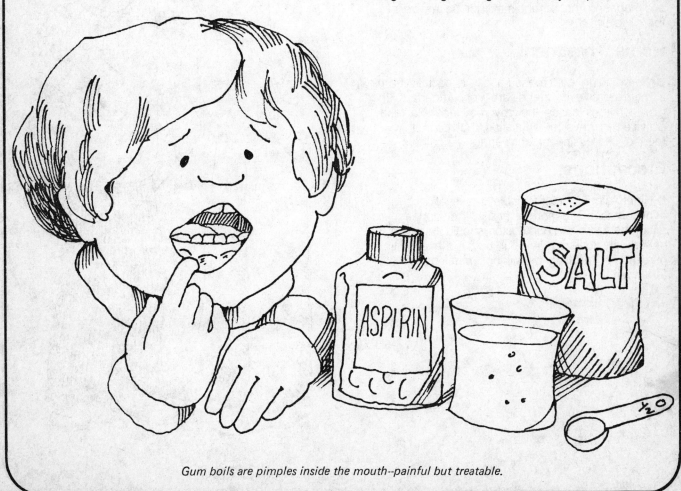

Gum boils are pimples inside the mouth--painful but treatable.

GYNECOMASTIA

Description

Gynecomastia is the development of breasts in a boy. Normal males have rudimentary breast tissue which can become enlarged by estrogens (female hormones) and rarely by androgens (male hormones). A boy with tumors of the testes or adrenal glands may develop appreciable breasts. Rarely, the same situation can occur from mistakenly ingesting sex hormones as medication or from eating poultry fattened by hormones.

Normal, adolescent boys commonly develop small breasts on one or both sides. These persist for two to twenty-four months, may be tender, and are often an embarrassment. The breasts may become quite pronounced and remain for years, but this is not common. Obese boys may develop large fat accumulations that resemble breasts (pseudogynecomastia) but which contain no true breast tissue.

Diagnosis

The diagnosis is obvious except when boys try to hide gynecomastia out of embarrassment. If this happens the parent may not be aware of the problem.

Home Treatment

Understanding and reassurance, especially from a male relative or friend, are very important. In more obvious cases the boy may need to take activities in physical education that do not require undressing or showering with others.

Precautions

• Ninety-eight percent of the cases of gynecomastia are normal and will disappear spontaneously. • Your doctor should have an opportunity to examine your boy if the condition persists. • Taunting by siblings must be firmly forbidden.

Doctor's Treatment

Your doctor will examine your boy carefully feeling for the presence or absence of true breast tissue, checking the coloration of areolae (nipples), and investigating abdominal or testicular masses and the distribution of sexual hair. A careful history of drug and food ingestion will be taken. If other causes of the condition are ruled out your doctor can only recommend your patience and support and counselling. Hormonal studies or chromosome studies are rarely needed. In severe or prolonged cases plastic surgery can remove breast tissue without visible scarring.

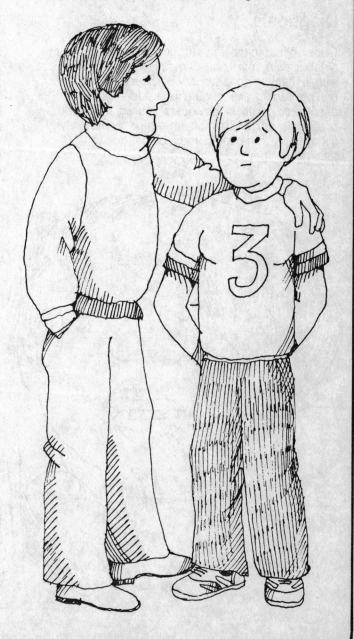

Gynecomastia calls for a man's understanding and support.

HAND, FOOT, & MOUTH DISEASE

Description

Hand, foot, and mouth disease is a common, easily recognizable, contagious illness caused by the coxsackie viruses. The disease is prevalent during warm weather and the average incubation period is three to five days. It is transmitted by contact with someone who has the disease (mouth-to-mouth) or by ingestion of fecally contaminated material.

The disease is characterized by blisters and sores in the mouth (cheeks, tongue, lips, throat) resembling canker sores, plus small clear blisters (one-sixteenth to one-eighth inch round) on the fingers, hands, toes, and feet. Fever may be absent, low (101°F), or high (104°F). Sometimes there is a viral rash on the skin. The illness lasts three to seven days.

Diagnosis

Typical appearance of the above symptoms is diagnostic. Other types of coxsackie illnesses in the family or among your child's friends are suggestive of the disease.

Home Treatment

Give aspirin or acetaminophen for fever and soreness of the mouth. Avoid foods that sting the mouth such as citrus juices, ginger ale, and spices. Administer antihistamines according to your doctor's directions if needed for the itchiness of blisters and rash.

Precautions

● This disease occasionally **can be dangerous for young infants.** Isolate babies from ill siblings. ● If your infant contracts this disease report it to your doctor.

Doctor's Treatment

Your doctor's treatment is the same as home treatment. Rarely will hospitalization of an ill and toxic infant for supportive therapy (relief of pain, intravenous feeding, etc.) be necessary.

Related Topics: Common Cold, Viruses

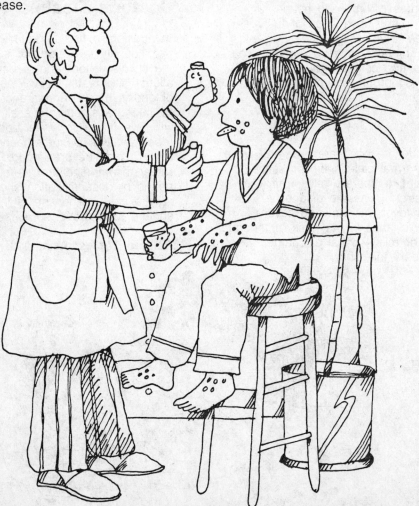

Aspirin or acetaminophen will reduce fever and relieve soreness.

HAY FEVER

Description

Hay fever is an allergic reaction of the membranes of the nose and sinuses to inhaled substances. When it occurs only during a particular time of the year (seasonal), hay fever is usually due to pollens of trees, grasses, or weeds. (Pollens of flowers are usually too heavy to be airborne or inhaled and are therefore seldom responsible.) When hay fever occurs year round (perennial) it may be due to dander from a cat, dog, horse, or cow (present in some felt underpaddings of carpeting) but rarely from guinea pigs, hamsters, gerbils, and mice. Feathers (pillows, comforters, and pet birds), house dust, and molds can also be responsible. Hay fever is rarely due to foods, beverages or medications.

Symptoms are nasal congestion, sneezing, clear nasal discharge, and itching of the nose which leads to the rubbing of the nose referred to as an "allergic salute." The eyes also may be involved. A headache results from involvement of sinuses. The ears feel obstructed and are sometimes painful, and hearing is diminished due to the obstruction of the eustachian tubes. Bluish bags under the eyes, called "allergic shiners," may be present. Your child may snore and complain of fatigue (allergic fatigue syndrome). In addition secondary bacterial infections are common.

Diagnosis

Membranes inside the nose are pale and white instead of the normal pink in the presence of hay fever. Prompt, temporary relief from oral antihistamines strengthens the diagnosis. Development of fever, moderate to severe earache, swollen glands in the neck, or opaque (green, yellow, or milky) nasal discharge indicates secondary infection.

Home Treatment

Consult your doctor concerning medications. Give oral antihistamines. Decongestants containing ephedrine, pseudoephedrine, or phenylpropanolamine may provide added relief. Reduce the child's exposure to offending substances (antigens) whenever possible. (The dander of a cat or dog allowed in the house only once a month can remain in the home for four to six weeks.) Keep the windows closed against pollens, and use an air conditioner if possible. Hot air ducts should have filters at room inlets to minimize dust. Use nonallergenic pillows and dehumidify the house.

Precautions

• Rubber pillows, which are considered nonallergenic, may breed molds as they age.
• Avoid repeated use of decongestant nose drops, which can cause worse congestion following the initial, brief relief.

Doctor's Treatment

In addition to home treatment your doctor can help identify the offending substance by taking the child's history and, if necessary, conducting allergy skin tests. He will substantiate the diagnosis by the appearance of the nose and by taking a smear of nasal secretions which will reveal allergic white blood cells (eosinophiles). Dexamethasone nasal spray (a steroid) may be prescribed. Your doctor will rarely recommend oral steroids for a brief period or desensitization shots for years for severe cases. The use of intranasal cromolyn sodium as a preventative is still experimental.

Related Topics: Asthma, Eye Allergies

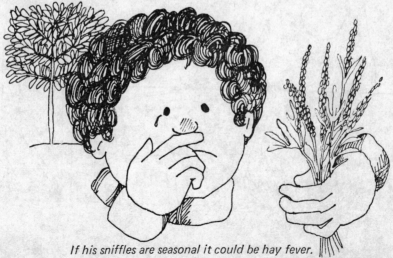

If his sniffles are seasonal it could be hay fever.

Description

Head lice are tiny parasites (smaller than fleas) less than one-eighth inch in length. They are grayish-white, almost transparent creatures with six legs. They live exclusively on humans, never on pets. They pass from one human to another and live on or close to the scalp where they bite and suck blood. Their visible eggs, which stick to the hairs, are milk-white and about the size of a flake of dandruff.

Head lice cause itching of the scalp and sometimes a red, scaly rash on the back of the neck at the hairline. Because of scratching, sores of the scalp may develop. The lymph glands at the base of the skull may be enlarged. During the past few years, infestation with head lice has become common among school-age children.

Diagnosis

Unless hundreds are present, it is difficult to see lice in a child's hair. Look for the small but easily visible eggs (called nits) attached to the shafts of the hairs. Nits are readily distinguished from flakes of dandruff which can be blown or brushed away; nits can scarcely be detached with fingernails.

Home Treatment

Apply two tablespoonfuls of a one percent gamma-benzene hexachloride shampoo (available by prescription) to your child's dry hair, work it into a lather, leave it on four minutes, then rinse. This kills both the lice and the eggs. Fine-comb your child's hair to remove the nits. If necessary a vinegar rinse will loosen the nits. Repeat the procedure once, four to seven days later. Clean combs and hairbrushes with gamma-benzene hexachloride shampoo. Clean hats and pillowcases by washing and ironing or by dry-cleaning to kill stray lice.

Lice can also be killed by the application of a 25-percent benzyl benzoate lotion (available over-the-counter) to the hair and scalp; shampoo after 12 to 24 hours. Repeat the procedure in four to seven days.

Precautions

● **Gamma-benzene hexachloride** is lindane, a white powder used chiefly as an insecticide, and **is poisonous** if swallowed or absorbed through the skin. Do not leave it within your child's reach. Do not apply it more than twice. ● If one person has head lice carefully check the heads of all other family members for evidence of infestation. ● If there are infected sores of the scalp or enlarged tender glands at the base of the skull consult your doctor.

Doctor's Treatment

Your doctor will treat head lice as you would at home. If there are infected sores and infected lymph glands your doctor may culture the sores and will usually prescribe an oral antibiotic for five to ten days.

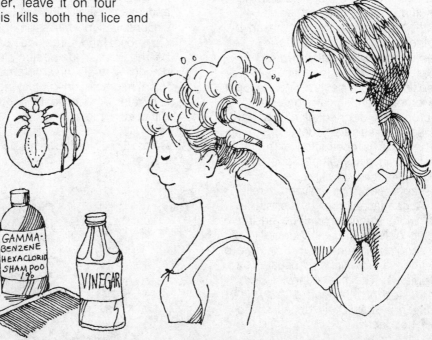

A medicated shampoo, followed by a vinegar rinse, will kill and remove both lice and nits.

HEADACHES

Description

Headaches are probably as common in children as in adults and have as many or more causes. Fever and strong emotions (anxiety, fear, excitement, sadness, and worry) account for 95 percent of all headaches. Less common causes are high blood pressure (hypertension), head injuries and concussions, tumors and infections of the brain (meningitis, encephalitis), bleeding inside the skull, sinusitis (allergic or infectious), eye strain, psychiatric problems, and epilepsy.

Diagnosis

The cause depends in large part upon a carefully detailed history and response to medications. In general a headache that responds to aspirin or acetaminophen—plus love—is not serious.

Migraine. A child that has a migraine usually has a strong family history of the condition. The headache is often one-sided and is generally accompanied by nausea and vomiting ("sick headache") and sometimes is preceded by an aura (seeing light flashes, or double vision etc.) It is most common in high achievers and self-motivated children. A migraine lasts for hours and usually responds poorly to aspirin and acetaminophen.

Hypertension. A throbbing pain occurs with a headache associated with hypertension. The child may sweat and turn pale or become flushed; heart and pulse pound. There is no relief from aspirin and acetaminophen.

Concussions. A concussion is diagnosed by history and other accompanying signs.

Tumor, infections, intracranial bleeding. Headaches associated with these illnesses become increasingly more severe and frequent. Vomiting and other neurological signs (stiff neck, visual problems, disorientation, loss of balance, and sometimes fever) develop.

Sinusitis. The nose is obstructed or runny when a child has sinusitis. Other signs of allergic rhinitis or infection are present. Antihistamines or nose drops may offer relief.

Eye strain. A headache from eye strain is never present while sleeping or upon arising. It parallels reading or watching television.

Psychiatric problems. Behavior problems are also present when a headache is caused by psychiatric problems. The headache is frequently at the top of the head or may affect the entire head, which is unusual with other forms of headache.

Home Treatment

Try aspirin, acetaminophen, antihistamines, or nose drops. Try reassurance, cuddling, and cold compresses. Lay the child down in a dark room. Try to remove any major family or school pressure from your child. If the headache persists see your doctor.

Precautions

• Sudden, severe headache—especially with fever, prostration, violent vomiting, disorientation or stiff neck—may be a **true emergency.** Get immediate, competent, professional advice. • Headaches that recur with increasing frequency and severity may be serious. See your doctor promptly. • Headaches with other neurological signs are almost always serious. See your doctor. • Investigation for cause of headaches may be simple or extremely complicated, but diagnosis depends heavily upon an accurate history. Observe the location of the pain, its duration, the time of day, the circumstances that provoke it, accompanying symptoms, and response to medications. Report these to your doctor.

Doctor's Treatment

Your doctor will perform a complete physical examination of your child, including measuring the blood pressure and examining the eyes (plus a neurological examination). Tests indicated are numerous and dictated by history and examination.

Consultation with a neurologist; allergist, ear, nose, and throat doctor; or psychiatrist may be required. Your doctor also may prescribe diagnostic trials of ergotamine and phenobarbital for a migraine. In perplexing cases your doctor can refer your child to a headache diagnostic clinic at a medical center.

Related Topics: Concussion, Hypertension

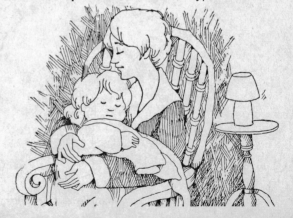

Cuddling and cold compresses can help your child's headache.

Description

Heat rash is the most common of all rashes in children of any age. Also known as prickly heat or miliaria, it is almost universal in babies during hot weather; heat rash can even occur in a cold climate if your child is overdressed either during the daytime or nighttime. Fair-skinned children (redheads and blonds) are the most frequent sufferers of heat rash, and they suffer the most from it. Usual locations are cheeks, neck, shoulders, skin creases, and diaper area. It frequently appears under wet bathing trunks.

Heat rash consists of hundreds of tiny pinhead eruptions each surrounding a skin pore. Those elements may be small, pink or red bumps or tiny water blisters. They are moderately itchy and may show scratch marks.

Diagnosis

History of exposure to hot humid conditions, perspiration, and overdressing are diagnostic clues. Diagnosis is confirmed by inspection of the rash with a magnifying glass in good light. Each dot of heat rash is seen at the mouth of a pore representing a sweat gland.

Home Treatment

Keep your child as cool as possible. If the heat rash is on your baby's face rest his face on an absorbent pad in the crib. Infants and children are safest from heat rash in an air-conditioned environment. Giving cool baths and sponging your child with diluted rubbing alcohol help. Baby powder or cornstarch applied lightly with a powder puff also helps. During warm weather, the use of prickly heat powders may give some relief. Give antihistamines by mouth if itching is intense.

Precautions

● Detergents and bleaches in clothing and bed linens may aggravate heat rash. ● Bubble baths, water softeners, and oily cosmetics should be avoided.

Doctor's Treatment

None.

Related Topic: Diaper Rash

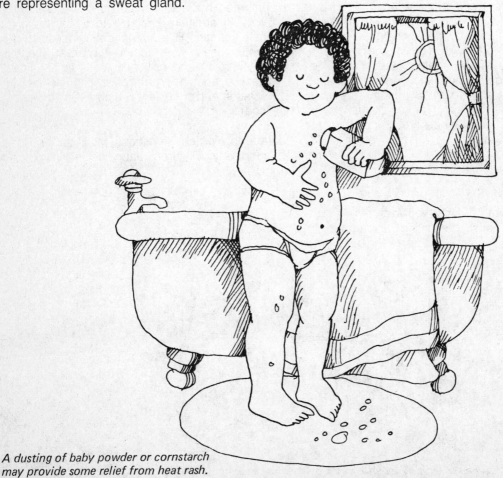

A dusting of baby powder or cornstarch may provide some relief from heat rash.

HEPATITIS

Description

Hepatitis is an infection of the liver. Only recently have the two causative viruses been identified. Hepatitis A virus causes infectious hepatitis. Hepatitis B virus causes serum hepatitis. Serious acute complications and chronic, progressive liver disease may occur with either form.

Hepatitis A is contracted from the stool or blood of a person with the disease. The virus is also present in contaminated water and food (for example, shellfish and milk). The incubation period is 15 to 45 days. The patient is contagious three weeks before the onset of jaundice until one week after onset. First symptoms are fever, malaise, headache, and sometimes the signs of common cold. Profound loss of appetite is an important early symptom. The liver is tender. After four to five days, jaundice appears (yellow skin and whites of eyes, dark amber urine, and light-colored stools). Jaundice lasts two to four weeks, followed by one to two months of diminishing fatigue.

Hepatitis B is contracted in one of two ways: either by close mouth-to-mouth contact or from the blood of a patient or carrier; it is transmitted usually by a blood transfusion or by an injection with a contaminated needle (as in drug addiction and tattooing). The incubation period is six weeks to six months. Hepatitis B is contagious during the incubation period and possibly for months and years. Symptoms are similar to hepatitis A but often more gradual and milder. Arthritis and rashes are common. Infectious mononucleosis can cause its own form of hepatitis.

Diagnosis

The striking symptoms are marked loss of appetite often with nausea, vomiting, and upper abdominal pain plus the onset of jaundice. The liver often is enlarged and tender. Specific diagnosis (A- or B-type) depends upon blood tests.

Home Treatment

If hepatitis is suspected, isolate your child from friends, school, or work to minimize the chance of contagion. Call your doctor. Home treatment consists of reasonable rest, liquids, and a low-fat diet.

Precautions

● If exposed, preventive gamma globulin or hepatitis B immune globulin injections must be given as soon after exposure as practical and before symptoms begin. ● If you must care for a child with hepatitis B remember that, contrary to past beliefs, this form is now known to be contagious. Practice good hygiene.

Doctor's Treatment

Your doctor may hospitalize your child for isolation as well as treatment. Diagnosis is confirmed by laboratory tests of the patient's blood. In addition available tests can determine when hepatitis B is no longer infectious. In severe cases, your doctor may treat hepatitis with steroids and oral antibiotics to sterilize the digestive tract and perform exchange transfusion (replacement of patient's blood with donor blood).

Related Topics: Infectious Mononucleosis, Jaundice in Children, Jaundice in Newborns

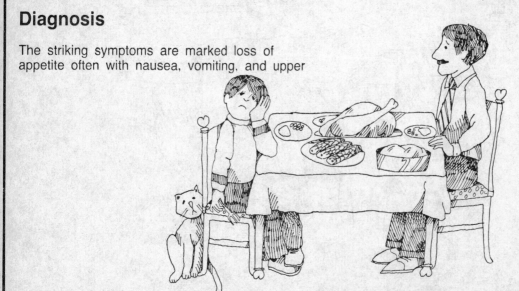

A marked loss of appetite is one of the most striking symptoms of hepatitis.

Description

A hernia, or rupture, is a protrusion of tissue through the wall of the body cavity. It might be compared to the protrusion of an inner tube through a hole in an automobile tire.

The most common hernia in a child is an *indirect inguinal hernia* which is always present but may or may not be detectable at birth. Usually, this form of hernia doesn't become apparent until some later age. It begins as a bulge just above the midpoint of the crease of the groin. It then enlarges toward the midline until it reaches and enters the scrotum of a boy or the labia majora of a girl. The bulge consists of a subcutaneous sac (peritoneum) which contains a portion of the omentum (a veil-like apron that overlies the intestines) or a loop of the small intestine. Less often, it contains a loop of the large bowel, urinary bladder, or ovary.

A rarer site is below the crease of the groin near where the pulse of the main artery to the leg can be felt. This is a *femoral hernia.* Infrequently, a true hernia appears in the midline of the abdomen above or below the navel as a *ventral hernia.* Frequently, a herniation is present at the umbilicus of infants and is called an *umbilical hernia.* This is not a true hernia, however, because it contains no sac, and it usually disappears spontaneously before age five.

Diagnosis

Diagnosis is made by the typical location and by noting that the contents of the sac can be pushed gently back (reduced) into the abdominal cavity. If a hernia cannot be reduced it is called incarcerated. If the blood supply to the contents of the hernia is cut off it is said to be strangulated. A strangulated hernia causes intense pain and swelling. Simple and incarcerated hernias produce no symptoms or merely a sense of heaviness.

Home Treatment

A hernia can be temporarily reduced by gentle pressure while the child is relaxed—in a warm tub if necessary. Trusses and belts to keep a hernia reduced are useless and may be harmful or even dangerous. Strapping an umbilical hernia is now considered of no benefit.

Precautions

● Strangulation of a hernia, with accompanying severe pain and sometimes nausea, vomiting, and prostration, is a **medical emergency** that requires immediate (within hours) surgical correction. ● Never attempt to reduce a strangulated hernia that has been present for more than a few minutes.

Doctor's Treatment

Surgical repair is required for all except umbilical hernias. An umbilical hernia usually cures itself. Although opinions vary as to the best time to correct a persistent umbilical hernia, the range is generally set from age two to age five or later. Since hernias often appear on both sides, the surgeon may correct both sides even though only one side is visibly herniated.

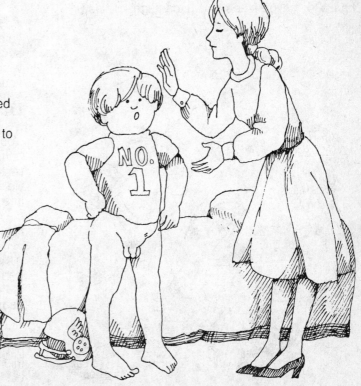

A hernia can become a medical emergency; watch it carefully.

HERPES SIMPLEX

Description

Herpes simplex is a highly contagious disease caused by herpesvirus hominis, types 1 and 2. Commonly called canker sores (in the mouth) or fever blisters (near the mouth), herpes simplex is transmitted by direct contact.

Infection with type 1 is common before age four but may occur at any age. It causes many painful ulcers of the membranes of the mouth (lips, cheeks, tongue, palate) and eyeballs; gums are red, swollen, and painful; the child's temperature may reach as high as 105°F; lymph nodes in the neck swell. The condition lasts seven to ten days. After the symptoms disappear, the virus continues to live in the body for months, years, or even throughout the individual's lifetime. When resistance is lowered by such conditions as fever, sunburn, exhaustion, or emotional stress, the "sleeping" virus is reactivated, and isolated, painful ulcers appear in or near the mouth or in a closely packed collection of small blisters on the skin. These are recurrent herpes and contagious.

Infection with type 2 herpesvirus hominis causes painful ulcers and blisters on the genitalia (labia, vagina, cervix, or penis). As with oral herpes, genital herpes is contagious and often recurrent. If a baby is delivered via the birth canal of a mother with genital herpes it can contract a generalized and overwhelming infection of herpesvirus and has a fifty percent chance of severe, permanent damage or death.

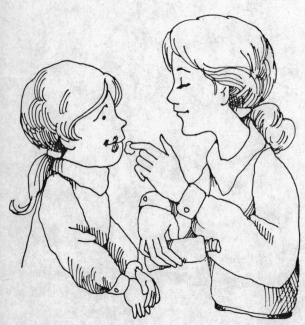

Apply antibiotic ointment to fever blisters to prevent cracking.

Diagnosis

The inital attack of herpes simplex is accompanied by fever, ulcers of the mouth, and swollen gums. Subsequent canker sores appear as open, red ulcers of the mouth which are unique in appearance. Gum boils protrude above the surface of the membranes; canker sores have a scooped-out appearance. Fever blisters are easily mistaken for impetigo but are generally more painful. To confuse the diagnosis, fever blisters may become secondarily infected with impetigo.

Home Treatment

Control pain and fever with aspirin or acetaminophen. Give bland, soothing foods such as ice cream, gelatin desserts, puddings, and milk. An older child may rinse his mouth with mild sodium perborate or table salt solutions. Canker sores can be treated with triamcinolone in dental ointment form or with thick solutions of local anesthetics available in brand-name form at your pharmacy. Application of antibiotic ointment to fever blisters may prevent painful cracking and stop impetigo from taking hold. (Some doctors recommend the application of ophthalmic solution of IDU—5-iodo-2' deoxyuridine—to fever blisters.)

Precautions

● Herpes simplex of the eyeball is serious. See your eye doctor promptly. ● Herpes can be severe in an infant. Keep siblings and adults with herpes from contact with the baby. See your doctor.

Doctor's Treatment

Your doctor will prescribe IDU eyedrops for herpes of the eyeball. Cytosine arabinoside (Ara-C) is an experimental drug available for life-threatening complications of herpes as in infants. A child with a severely ulcerated mouth may require hospitalization and intravenous fluids until he is able to swallow liquids.

If a mother who is about to deliver has genital herpes, a Cesarean section may be performed within four hours of the rupture of maternal membranes to avoid exposing the baby to the disease. The newborn must then be isolated from the mother.

There is no way to eradicate recurrent herpes. Repeated smallpox vaccinations and injections of vitamins are not effective and may be harmful.

Related Topics: Gum Boils, Impetigo

Description

Children are prone to joint pains, most of which are transitory and not serious (sprains, growing pains). Occasionally arthritis appears in children. In addition, there are three specific causes of pain in the hip that are common and must be differentiated.

Acute synovitis of the hip. This condition may be thought of as a bruise of the inside of the hip joint. It may be caused by injuries which are often trivial, like those caused by jumping, for instance. It can occur at any age but most frequently happens between ages two and six. Acute synoritis is almost always a benign, self-curing condition. Fever (low-grade if present) is rare.

Legg-Calvé-Perthes disease. This serious condition of the hip is of unknown origin. The upper end of the thigh bone (femoral head) softens and becomes deformed. The onset of the condition is usually between ages four and ten years, and most often affects boys. It is rarely on both sides. If untreated Legg-Calvé-Perthes disease results in a permanent, severe deformity of the hip. Fever is absent.

Slipped femoral epiphysis. The cause of this condition is unknown, but possibly it is a delayed result of injury. It primarily occurs during the teen years and usually to overweight (obese or muscular) child. Severe deformity results if it is untreated. Fever is absent.

Diagnosis

All three conditions cause a pain in the hip with an accompanying limp. A child may complain of knee pain when the origin of the pain is in the hip. The hip joint is limited in one or more of its movements: flexion and extension, inward and outward rotation, and adduction and abduction (movement toward and away from the midline).

Home Treatment

Keep your child off his legs for three to four days. Crawling instead of walking does not keep weight off the hip. If the condition is not cured see your doctor.

Precautions

● If your child has pain in his knee he may have a hip disease. Examine his hip whenever your child complains of knee pains. ● Marked pain, limp, and high fever may be a serious form of arthritis. Consult your doctor.

Doctor's Treatment

Your doctor's careful examination may include an X ray of the hips. However, Legg-Calvé-Perthes disease and slipped epiphysis do not always show up on first X rays, and synovitis rarely shows at all. Your doctor may suggest that your child continue bed rest, in or out of the hospital. Traction may be prescribed in the hospital, and X rays may be taken at intervals so your doctor may carefully follow the progress of treatment. Tests for arthritis may also be performed. Slipped epiphysis is always treated by surgery. Legg-Calvé-Perthes disease sometimes requires surgery and is treated by keeping the weight off the legs and forbidding walking for many months until the condition heals.

Related Topics: Arthritis, Growing Pains, Knee Pains, Sprains and Dislocations

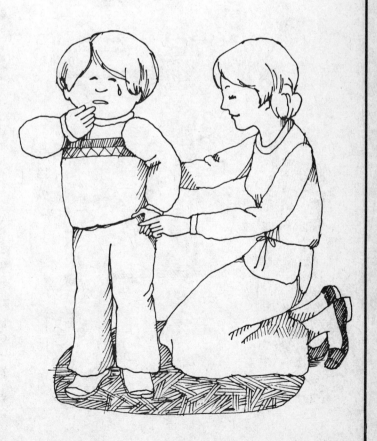

Pain in the hip accompanied by a limp should be checked out carefully.

HIVES

Description

Hives (urticaria) are an allergic reaction of the skin. Hives appear as red, itchy, raised welts that range in size from one-fourth inch to several inches in diameter. Twenty percent of children have hives once or repeatedly. Hives may involve any area of skin. They often result in huge swelling of the genitalia and swelling of the lips of the mouth. Their most characteristic aspect is their rapidly changing appearance—hives come and go and change size hourly.

Ninety-five percent of the cases are caused by ingestion of foods, beverages, or medications to which the child is allergic. Citrus fruits, chocolate, nuts (peanut butter), tomatoes, berries, spices, candies, tropical fruits (juices), and artificial flavorings are particular offenders. The remaining five percent of cases are caused by something the child has come in contact with (e.g., plants, ointments, cosmetics, dog and cat saliva), insect bites and stings, excessive exposure to the sun or cold, or inhalants (e.g., pollens, insecticides, molds, animal dander, feathers). An unusual form of hives is caused by respiratory and other viruses, medications, and streptococcus. This form is called *erythema multiforme* and looks like different-sized red targets painted on the skin. Hives sometimes cause allergic arthritis.

Diagnosis

All welts that itch and rapidly change appearance are hives. No other rash has these traits. An insect bite is hive-like at the point of the bite, but it does not come and go rapidly. Hives that are caused by an allergy to insects are at sites distant from the bite.

Home Treatment

To pinpoint the cause consider your child's activities during the minutes or hours preceding the onset of hives. Oral antihistamines usually work well and may have to be continued for up to a week if hives recur. Cold applications, calamine lotion, and cornstarch baths may be of some help.

Precautions

● If hives involve the tongue or cause a cough or difficulty in breathing or swallowing see your doctor **immediately**. ● If hives are accompanied by fever see your doctor to rule out strep infections. ● If antihistamines don't help telephone your doctor for advice.

Doctor's Treatment

Your doctor may administer epinephrine and Sus-Phrine bronchodilator and decongestants, steroids, or antihistamines by injection if the case is severe. Oral steroids will be tried if antihistamines are ineffective. If hives are recurrent and the cause is not clear from your child's history your doctor may perform skin tests or refer your child to an allergist. A throat culture may be ordered to check for strep infection. If symptoms of arthritis are present your doctor may order tests for confirmation of the disorder. If hives are caused by insects your doctor will probably suggest a long-term course (years) of desensitizing shots. In such a case your child should carry medications with him to take if he is stung.

Calamine lotion can soothe the itch of hives.

Related Topic: Arthritis

Description

Any condition that interferes with the normal vibrations of the vocal cords can produce hoarseness. Extreme hoarseness causes a total voice loss.

The most common cause of hoarseness in children is abuse of the voice (i.e. screaming) that results in swelling of the vocal cords and hoarseness. If hoarseness occurs frequently, tiny wart-like growths form on the cords to produce chronic hoarseness. The growths are called "singer's nodes" in adults and "screamer's nodes" in children. Other causes of hoarseness in children are croup, laryngitis, and allergies. Rarer causes are diphtheria, foreign bodies that have been inhaled, and injuries of the larynx.

Babies are sometimes born with soft larynxes that partially collapse with each inhalation, causing a crowing sound (*congenital laryngeal stridor*). This condition may impart a hoarseness to your infant's cry.

Diagnosis

If your child speaks or cries in a lower pitch than usual or refuses to speak above a whisper, the cause is diagnosed by history and by the presence or absence of other symptoms (fever, cough, difficult breathing, sore throat, nasal obstruction).

Home Treatment

Persuade your child to rest his voice. Inhalation of steam and drinking warm liquids are helpful. A warm application to the neck is an old remedy that works. If an allergy is present, give your child antihistamines. Congenital laryngeal stridor is self-curing by age one year.

Precautions

● If other signs of illness are absent, hoarseness is non-threatening and may be ignored. Malignancies that can cause hoarseness in children are virtually unknown.
● If hoarseness worsens day by day or persists unchanged beyond a month, consult your doctor.

Doctor's Treatment

A doctor using a tongue blade and flashlight can see no deeper than the epiglottis, which is above the vocal cords, but experienced ear, nose, and throat specialists can see the vocal cords with mirrors and other instruments. Hoarseness often responds to a course of oral steroids if the return of the voice to normal is urgent. Surgery is rarely indicated for removal of "screamers' nodes."

Related Topics: Choking, Croup, Diphtheria, Laryngitis

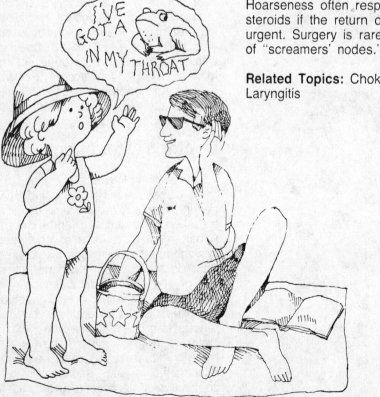

Feed a "frog" warm liquids to ease it away.

HYPERACTIVITY

Description

All healthy children are active. Most are more active at least part of the time than a sedate adult would prefer and some are very active. Of these active children only one to ten percent have true hyperkinesis, a condition in which (under most circumstances) they are unable to be quiet and motionless for more than a few moments.

Hyperactivity (hyperkinesis) is part of the clinical picture described as minimal brain dysfunction (MBD). Other symptoms that may be present in any combination are: poor coordination (clumsiness), emotional outbursts, lack of concentration, and learning disabilities. Hyperactivity may be due to late or faulty development of the brain centers whose functions are to filter incoming stimuli (sights, sounds, smells, touches, tastes) and to regulate self-control. Behavior that closely mimics hyperactivity is seen in children with normal brain centers, but whose centers were never stimulated or taught. Children raised in total permissiveness or neglect may have such untutored control centers.

Diagnosis

Hyperactivity is fairly obvious in extreme cases: the child is constantly in physical motion. This behavior is annoying and often destructive, but not malicious. The child cannot sit still to be read to or in front of a television screen for more than a few seconds or minutes.

Most cases are less severe and consequently more difficult to diagnose. Check with school officials and your physician concerning your child's legal right to evaluation and treatment. Testing by a trained psychologist is often necessary. Neurological examination and an electroencephalogram are universally recommended by non-medical professionals (e.g. educators), but rarely are of diagnostic help. An experienced neurologist may recognize a hyperkinetic child at a glance.

Home Treatment

Home treatment is limited without professional advice. Once professional advice has been obtained, home treatment is of great importance but only as it is tailored to a particular child's needs. Caffeine (strong coffee) sometimes lessens hyperkinesis, but is not advised without professional advice. The avoidance of all foods with artificial colorings, flavorings, and preservatives is reputed to help. However, the special attention required to maintain such a diet may account for any improvement in the child's behavior.

Precautions

● True hyperactivity is present from infancy. If your normally behaved child suddenly becomes overactive past the age of one or two years, look for clues in the child's environment. ● If your child is overactive with one parent and not with the other the child does not have hyperkinesis. ● Only accept a decision concerning hyperactivity from an experienced, trained, and skilled profesional. Accurate diagnosis often requires a team approach.

Doctor's Treatment

Your doctor will give a complete physical and neurological examination, including vision and hearing tests. A careful and detailed history will be taken, and school reports will be evaluated. A battery of tests by a psychologist (psychometrics) will generally be recommended. Your doctor may try a diagnostic or therapeutic trial of stimulant medications (dextro-amphetamine, methylphenidate, pemoline), and will require accurate follow-up reports from parents and teachers regarding any changes in your child's behavior. The hyperkinetic child will often need special educational facilities and sometimes psychiatric counseling for emotional problems which are secondary to his poor family, peer, and school relationships.

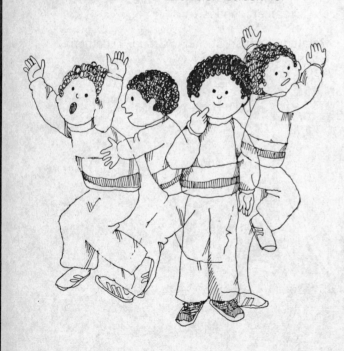

The truly hyperactive child cannot sit still.

Description

Although it's been known for decades. many people are still unaware that hypertension (high blood pressure) occurs in children and in infants as well as adults. Normal blood pressure at birth is about 80/40 millimeters of mercury; systolic over diastolic. The blood pressure then gradually rises until in adolescence it is approximately 120/80. Substantial elevation above these figures should be evaluated.

The most common cause of hypertension is apprehension. (Diastolic pressure is little or not at all elevated.) Other causes of hypertension in children are: kidney disease (tumors, obstructions, infections, nephritis); adrenal and testicular tumors; congenital defects of the heart or a major artery (coarctation of aorta); hyperactive thyroid; "essential hypertension" (the most common cause in adults, which may be hereditary); medications (steroids, ephedrine); extreme obesity; and, curiously, excessive eating of licorice. Hypertension may cause headaches, pounding heartbeat, shortness of breath during exercise, and flushing of the face.

Diagnosis

Diagnosis must be made by careful blood pressure measurements at each annual physical examination, using proper size instruments commensurate with your child's age. If the blood pressure is elevated once it must be taken one or more times at short intervals to be sure of the reading before starting an investigation of the cause.

Home Treatment

None. An annual physical examination is recommended. Virtually all hypertensions of childhood are curable but can be dangerous if not treated.

Precautions

● Be sure your doctor includes blood pressure measurement during the annual physical.

Doctor's Treatment

Your doctor will give a complete physical examination including blood pressure, palpation of arteries in the groin, and examination of eyegrounds (where results of hypertension may appear early), heart, abdomen, and genitalia.

Laboratory investigation of confirmed hypertension is complicated and involves checking all the causes listed above. The condition frequently requires hospitalization. Except for rare cases, all causes can be successfully treated or cured by medications, changes in diet, or surgery.

Related Topics: Nephritis, Thyroid

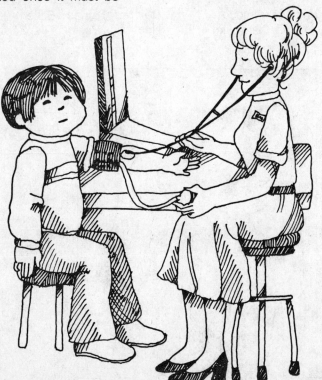

Be sure your child's blood pressure is measured at each annual physical.

IMPETIGO

Description

Impetigo is a highly contagious infection of the superficial layers of the skin. It is caused by staphylococcus and/or streptococcus germs. It is transmitted by direct contact with infected persons or objects such as clothing, towels, toys, and sandboxes. The incubation period is two to five days.

Impetigo typically starts as a fragile blister containing thin, yellow pus. The blister is easily broken, leaving an open, weeping sore that increases in size. The discharge hardens into a yellow crust or scab and readily spreads the disease to other areas of the skin. The initial sore is often at the point of injured skin, which has been irritated by an insect bite, scrape, poison ivy, eczema, or (around the nostrils) from picking the nose. If the infecting germ is caused by streptococcus, glomerulonephritis—a kidney complication—may develop.

Diagnosis

Rapidly spreading, moist sores that form crusts that resemble hardened honey are characteristic of impetigo. Any open wound that fails to heal promptly should suggest impetigo. Distinction between streptococcal and staphylococcal infection can be made only by a culture.

Home Treatment

If only a few small areas are involved remove the crusts of the lesions by softening them with soap and water. (Streptococcal and staphylococcal infections thrive *under* the crusts.) Apply an antibiotic ointment several times daily. Cover the sores with gauze to keep the ointment in place and to discourage your child from scratching and spreading the disease.

Precautions

● Treat minor scratches and scrapes with soap and water and a sterile bandage to avoid impetigo. ● If your child has impetigo watch the rest of the family carefully and treat cases promptly if they occur. ● Keep the wash cloth, towel, and clothing used by a child with impetigo separate from others' items to reduce the chance of it spreading. Ordinary laundering adequately sterilizes clothing. ● If home treatment is not promptly effective see your doctor. ● Do not discontinue treatment that is working until the sores are completely healed and the skin is smooth. Eradication may require extended treatment.

Doctor's Treatment

Your doctor may culture sores and prescribe penicillin for ten to fourteen days if streptococcal infection is present. Sensitivity tests on a staphylococcal infection may be required to determine the most effective antibiotic.

Related Topics: Eczema, Insect Bites, Nephritis, Poison Ivy, Scrapes

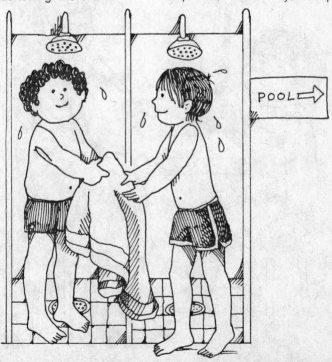

Impetigo, highly contagious, can be transmitted through contact with infected towels and clothing.

INFECTIOUS MONONUCLEOSIS

Description

Infectious mononucleosis is a common, contagious disease caused by Epstein-Barr (EB) virus. It most often occurs among those of secondary-school and college age, but it can occur at any age from infancy on. The disease is transmitted via droplets from the nose and throat; it is popularly known as "the kissing disease." The incubation period is one to six weeks, long enough to have forgotten whom you kissed. One attack usually gives lifelong immunity.

The usual symptoms of "mono" are malaise, sore throat, prolonged fever, and a generalized swelling of the lymph glands, which are barely or not at all tender. Ten to twenty percent of the cases have a nonspecific, red, mottled rash, especially on the trunk. Acute illness may last for weeks; fatigue and weakness may go on for months. Complications of mono are hepatitis, ruptured spleen, encephalitis, and spontaneous bleeding (purpura).

Diagnosis

Because mono symptoms suggest other diseases, diagnosis is rarely possible without laboratory tests. Fever, severe sore throat (often with pus or gray membrane on the tonsils), swollen neck glands, and rash, may suggest strep throat, tonsillitis, or diphtheria. However, the failure of the symptoms to improve with time and treatment raises the suspicion of mononucleosis. Enlargement of the spleen and lymph nodes, plus bruised-looking areas of the skin or mucous membranes may raise unfounded fears of leukemia.

Complications like encephalitis or hepatitis with jaundice may make the diagnosis more difficult.

Home Treatment

Rest, aspirin or acetaminophen, and diet as tolerated are indicated. If the spleen is enlarged, your child should be prevented from participating in contact sports or other violent activity until the spleen returns to its normal size to avoid rupture. This may take weeks or months. (An enlarged spleen protrudes beneath the ribs which normally protect it and it is vulnerable to injury and rupture.) Although mono is contagious, isolation is not required. Your child may return to school as soon as weakness and fatigue subside. Secondary cases in a family are rare.

Rest, aspirin, and proper diet are important parts of hom treatment for infectious mononucleosis.

Precautions

● Ten to twenty percent of the cases of mono have a positive throat culture for streptococcal infection for which antibiotic therapy is required. If your child, ill and with a positive throat culture, does not improve promptly (within 24 to 48 hours) in response to the prescribed antibiotic, report to your doctor so that tests for infectious mononucleosis can be done.

Doctor's Treatment

Your doctor will give your child a complete physical examination including evaluation of the liver, spleen, and all lymph node sites. Your doctor also will perform a throat culture. A blood count may reveal white blood cells characteristic of mononucleosis (Downy cells). A positive blood test for heterophile antibody level helps confirm diagnosis. Unfortunately, a blood count and heterophile test may be normal at the beginning of the illness and, in rare cases, may remain nondiagnostic throughout the illness.

A course of oral steroid therapy promptly relieves all symptoms except those caused by complications. Although medical educators disagree, steroids should be given unless a specific condition prohibits their use such as gastric ulcer, hypertension, or aneurysm. If the throat culture is positive for streptococcal infection, penicillin or other antibiotic therapy is indicated. Severe cases require hospitalization for the administration of intravenous fluids, possible transfusions, and for supportive treatment.

Related Topics: Diphtheria, Encephalitis, Hepatitis, Lymph Nodes—Infection Fighters, Strep Throat, Tonsillitis

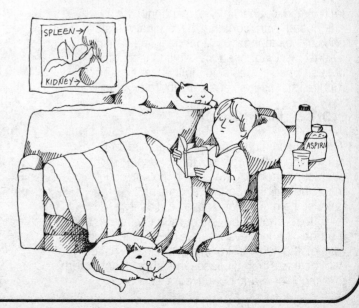

INFLUENZA

Description

Any viral infection of the upper respiratory tract is apt to be referred to as "flu," particularly if it is accompanied by chills, fever, cough, and muscle aches. Influenza is, however, a highly contagious, *specific* respiratory infection which occurs in epidemics and is caused by the influenza A or influenza B virus. It is transmitted by droplets from nose and throat discharges of persons who have the disease. It has a short incubation period of one to three days and is contagious for seven days starting before symptoms appear.

The symptoms are: sudden chills, a sharp rise in body temperature to 102°F to 106°F (sometimes with febrile convulsion), flushing, headache, sore throat, a hacking cough, redness of the eyes, and pains in the back and limbs. In young children vomiting and diarrhea may occur. Fever lasts three to four days and is followed by days of weakness and fatigue during which the child is vulnerable to other illnesses.

Secondary bacterial complications are responsible for many of the serious outcomes of flu, and their presence is suggested by: the return of high fever after the third or fourth day of normal temperature; progressive worsening of the cough changing from dry and hacking to loose and productive; formation of pus in the eyes or a change in nasal discharge from clear to thick and yellow; rapid breathing and shortness of breath beyond that expected from the fever; severe earache; stiff neck; disorientation; and the onset of prostration.

Diagnosis

In isolated cases, influenza cannot be diagnosed with certainty by ordinary tests or on physical examination. During an epidemic. the disease is diagnosed by similarity to other cases. Specific tests for influenza viruses require the use of special laboratory facilities.

Home Treatment

The "prescription" for home care is: bed rest during the height of the fever; aspirin or acetaminophen for fever and pains: cough medicines if the cough is causing fatigue, pain, or sleep loss. Fluids—as tolerated—should be encouraged to clear toxins through the kidneys. Isolate your child from the rest of the family. To minimize the probability of contracting other diseases he should not return to school or work during convalescence.

Precautions

● Watch for signs of complications and report their occurrence to your doctor. ● Without complications the fever associated with influenza often peaks in two cycles (diphasic). It is elevated for a day or two, normal for a day, and elevated for a day or two. Do not misinterpret 24 hours of normal temperature as a "cure," and do not allow your child to resume activities until his temperature is normal for two or more days and he is feeling well.

Doctor's Treatment

Your doctor's treatment is the same as home treatment. Antibiotics, cultures, blood count, and possibly hospitalization may be required to treat complications.

Preventative vaccines have limited usefulness in children. Influenza viruses frequently mutate (spontaneously change their structure) from year to year, and last year's vaccine may be useless against this year's virus. Moreover, reactions to influenza vaccines in children are frequent though rarely serious. The current thinking is that only children at special risk from influenza should have annual immunization and then only with a "split virus" vaccine that causes few reactions. The conditions that constitute special risks are: rheumatic heart disease, congenital and hypertensive heart disease, cystic fibrosis, severe asthma, tuberculosis, nephrosis, chronic nephritis, chronic diseases of the nervous system, and diabetes.

Related Topics: Common Cold, Convulsions with Fever, Coughs, Fever

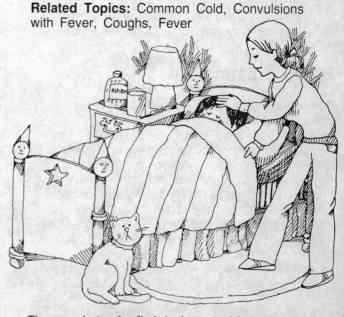

The prescription for flu is bed rest, aspirin, and isolation.

INGROWN TOENAILS

Description

The corners and edges of toenails may break the skin surrounding the nail. Once the skin is broken, conditions exist that encourage chronic infection. The infection causes the tissues to swell, further embedding the corner of the nail. The toe becomes red, painful, and tender to the touch, and thin, watery pus is discharged from the wound and works its way under the nail. This condition is known as ingrown toenail, and no healing is possible as long as the nail remains within the wound.

The initial wound may be caused by injury to the toe as a result of being stepped on or squeezed by ill-fitting shoes. Or the nail may have been trimmed in a manner that creates a sharp spur at the corner that pierces the skin like a dagger as the nail grows.

Most cases of ingrown toenails involve the big toes of older children but any toe can be involved. A baby can develop an ingrown toenail by digging his bare toes into the mat of the crib or other surface where he has been placed face down.

Diagnosis

There should be no mistake in recognizing the gradually worsening tenderness, redness, pain, and swelling that eventually involves one entire side of a toenail. Often the nail becomes partly covered by raw, red tissue (granulation tissue) and a wet crust.

Home Treatment

Recognized early, an ingrown toenail can be successfully treated by gently cutting out the spur or the ingrown corner of the nail and then soaking the toe for a long time. Even if the embedded nail cannot be removed because of the tenderness proper and prolonged soaking in a strong Epsom salts solution (one cup to one quart of water) may cure the condition. Cover the lower foot and toe with a bandage or cloth, soak thoroughly in the solution, and cover the dripping foot with plastic wrapping or encase the foot in a plastic bag. In this manner the nail can be soaked for hours with little effort, even overnight or for a number of days if necessary. Because of the delicacy of the nails involved, the ingrown toenails of infants can often be cured by wiping them several times a day with rubbing alcohol.

Precautions

● If your child repeatedly develops ingrown toenails check for shoes that are too small or too pointed. ● Check your child's method of trimming his toenails. ● An infection near the nail that lasts for more than a few days is probably an ingrown nail.

Doctor's Treatment

Your doctor's treatment will often be the same as home treatment, although your doctor is able to use a local anesthetic to remove the embedded nail and do a more thorough job. If ingrown toenails frequently occur your doctor may suggest minor surgery that permanently narrows the nail and makes ingrowing less likely.

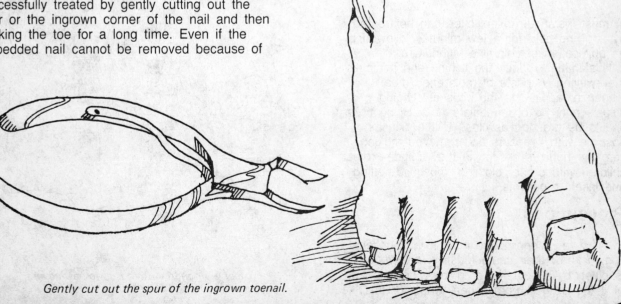

Gently cut out the spur of the ingrown toenail.

INSECT BITES

Description

The bites and stings of most insects are minor annoyances to most children. The only common complication is impetigo from scratching. Insect bites can cause serious illnesses.

Black widow spiders and *scorpions* can inject a venom potent enough to kill.

The *brown recluse spider* bite can cause a large sloughing ulcer and fever.

Female wood tick bites can cause an ascending paralysis and death.

Bees, wasps, hornets, and yellow jackets can cause severe reactions in persons who are allergic—generalized hives, asthma, circulatory collapse, and death (anaphylaxis).

Some children become sensitized (allergic) to the bites of mosquitoes, stable flies, fleas, and lice, but the allergic reactions are usually less severe than those caused by stinging insects.

Among diseases transmitted by insect bites are Rocky Mountain spotted fever, Colorado tick fever, and tularemia (wood ticks), rickettsialpox (mouse mites), viral encephalitis (mosquitoes), and typhus (red mites, lice and rat fleas).

Diagnosis

Flying insects usually bite only exposed areas of the skin. Crawling insects bite anywhere and often in groups. Flea bites tend to concentrate on the ankles and lower legs. Bedbug bites are often three to five bites arranged in a relatively straight line, an inch or two apart. Honeybees leave the stinger in the bite; bumblebees and other stinging insects do not. Ticks remain attached to the skin for long periods while biting, and resemble small plump raisins.

Home Treatment

In most instances insect bites can be treated by applying cold for a few minutes followed by an application of calamine lotion. Oral antihistamines reduce the itching and minimize the swelling. A paste of moistened meat tenderizer applied to the bites of stinging insects may be of immediate help. Biting ticks should be grasped as close to the skin as possible with tweezers and removed making sure the head is not left in the wound. Protect children with proper clothing, mosquito-netting, and insect repellents.

Precautions

● Learn to recognize the insects in your locale and to know their characteristics. ● If your child is bitten by a scorpion or black widow spider, or if the sting is from a bee, wasp, or the like and the child develops hives, or breathing, speaking, or swallowing is difficult, place a tourniquet above the bite and proceed to the nearest medical facility.*

Doctor's Treatment

Allergic reactions are treated with epinephrine, antihistamines, or steroids. A child who is allergic should have desensitizing injections. Also, your doctor may prescribe a kit for immediate home treatment.

Your doctor will give antivenom for use against scorpion and black widow spider bites and will administer steroids for these and for brown recluse spider bites.

Related Topics: Hives, Impetigo, Rocky Mountain Spotted Fever

*Current thinking is that a tourniquet, once put on, should be left on, not loosened and tightened as instructions once indicated, and the patient rushed to the medical facility.

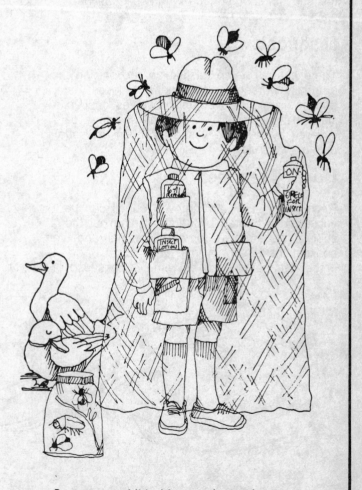

Protect your child with mosquito netting and insect repellents.

INTESTINAL ALLERGIES

Description

Infants are the most likely sufferers of intestinal allergies. The condition involves vomiting, diarrhea, and abdominal cramps and occurs from minutes to hours after the child has ingested certain foods, beverages, or medications. The most common offending food is nonpasteurized cow's milk; but eggs, wheat, soybean formulas, orange juice, tomatoes, chocolate, fish, berries, and melons may also be responsible. Sometimes, blood may be seen in the stools; other signs include hives, eczema, runny nose, and asthma.

Resembling the symptoms of an intestinal allergy but not allergies at all are the malabsorption syndromes which result in "failure to thrive." A malabsorption syndrome arises from an enzyme deficiency. Normally, the intestines and the pancreas produce enzymes that break down starches, fats, proteins and sugars. In a malabsorption syndrome, an enzyme is missing, and certain foods cannot be digested. For example, celiac disease may interfere with the digestion of gluten (starch found in wheat and rye), and cystic fibrosis may hamper the digestion of fats and proteins.

Diagnosis

If a particular food brings on abdominal cramps and diarrhea (with or without vomiting), an intestinal allergy or malabsorption syndrome can be suspected. By judiciously changing the diet and observing your child's physical reactions, you may make a preliminary diagnosis. Often, however, specific and complex tests are required.

Home Treatment

If your infant begins to vomit or has cramps or diarrhea after a new food has been introduced into his diet, stop the food promptly. Add new foods one at a time and allow several days between each introduction.

Precautions

● Persistent diarrhea is a clue to a malabsorption or an allergic problem. Broad-spectrum antibiotics and gastrointestinal viruses may cause a temporary loss of digestive enzymes, particularly lactase (the enzyme that digests milk sugar). ● Temporarily eliminate milk and milk products if diarrhea persists. ● Symptoms of malabsorption call for a sweat test to rule out cystic fibrosis.

Doctor's Treatment

Doctors diagnose these maladies on the basis of: dietary changes; culture and examination of stools for blood, fat, and starch; analysis of digestive enzymes; biopsy of the intestinal lining; sugar (lactose, glucose, and xylose) tolerance tests; sweat test; chest X rays; and other factors. Treatment involves dietary control and, sometimes, a prescription of digestive enzyme supplements.

Related Topic: Cystic Fibrosis

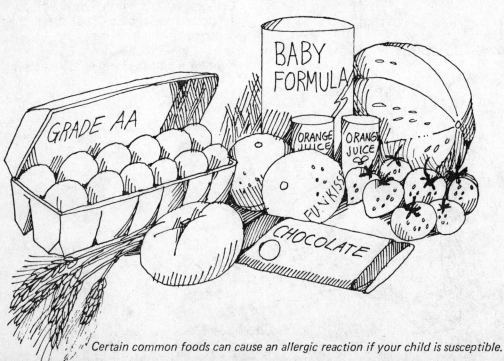

Certain common foods can cause an allergic reaction if your child is susceptible.

JAUNDICE IN CHILDREN

Description

Jaundice is a yellowing of the skin and the whites of the eyes due to the accumulation of bilirubin in the body. When a child has jaundice, all of the body fluids are stained; the tears are yellow, and the urine is dark orange.

Bilirubin comes from the hemoglobin that is released when old red blood cells are replaced by new cells. It is excreted by the liver into the intestine as bile. Jaundice develops when the red blood cells are rapidly destroyed (as in sickle cell, Mediterranean, spherocytic and other, rarer forms of anemia); when the liver cannot transform bilirubin into bile; or when bile cannot flow through the bile ducts into the intestines. Certain medications, including chlorpromazine (an antinauseant) and erythromycin estolate,

may temporarily impede the function of the liver and bring on jaundice. Blockage of the bile ducts by stones, cysts, or congenital malformation can also provoke jaundice. The disease may be caused by some drugs and poisons and is rarely the complication of a more generalized infection.

The usual cause of jaundice in children over one month of age is hepatitis. Damage to the liver cells by the hepatitis virus interferes with the formation of bile.

Diagnosis

The yellow-gold-orange color of the skin and whites of the eyes suggests jaundice. However, the diagnosis can be exceedingly complex and depends upon laboratory tests.

Home Treatment

Only after a clear diagnosis has been made can anything be done in the home. Then, antihistamines may lessen the itching of jaundice.

Precautions

● Jaundice caused by medication stops when the drugs are stopped. Other causes of jaundice in children are potentially serious and hard to diagnose. They all require a doctor's attention.

Doctor's Treatment

Doctors usually hospitalize children with suspected jaundice to treat the problem and to conduct laboratory tests.

Related Topics: Hepatitis, Jaundice In Newborns

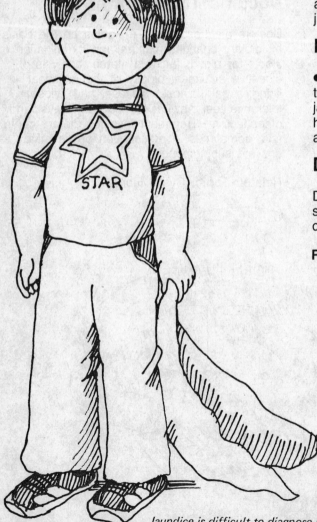

Jaundice is difficult to diagnose and requires a doctor's attention.

Description

Because a newborn infant's nervous system is vulnerable to permanent damage, jaundice during the first days of life has special significance. Jaundice occurs in infants due to an excessive breakdown of red blood cells or to the liver's inability to rapidly remove bilirubin from the blood.

Sixty percent of full-term infants and eighty percent of premature babies develop a normal jaundice during the first week of life. This occurs due to the rapid destruction of the excess number of red blood cells with which all healthy babies are born. It usually begins on the second or third day of life and disappears between the fifth and tenth day. With rare exceptions, this jaundice is harmless. It's major importance is the difficulty it presents in being distinguished from abnormal jaundice.

The two most frequent causes of abnormal jaundice in the newborn are erythroblastosis fetalis and sepsis (blood poisoning). Erythroblastosis fetalis is due to an incompatibility between the blood of the child and the mother. The mismatch may be in the Rh factor (for example, when the mother is Rh-negative but the infant is Rh-positive) or in the ABO factors (when the mother is type O but the baby is type B) or in rarer blood factors. Because of the incompatibility, the mother forms antibodies that rapidly destroy the infant's red blood cells. Sepsis (a generalized infection caused by bacteria or viruses) causes jaundice in the newborn by destroying red blood cells and injuring the liver.

Breast-fed newborns may also develop jaundice because a substance in the mother's milk interferes with the function of the liver. This form of jaundice by itself usually is harmless. There are scores of other causes of jaundice in the newborn, including congenital anemias (Cooley's, spherocytic, sickle cell), hepatitis, and German measles, but they are rare.

Diagnosis

Because erythroblastosis fetalis and sepsis can be fatal to newborn babies if not treated immediately, a doctor's diagnosis must be made promptly. Other forms of jaundice can also be serious if the bilirubin in the blood exceeds a safe level. In suspected cases of jaundice, a doctor must monitor the bilirubin level closely.

Home Treatment

Parents, it is your responsibility to watch out for the development of jaundice in the first week of your child's life at home. To judge the yellowness of the skin and eyes accurately, observe the baby in natural light. (Artificial light obscures the true color.)

Precautions

● Jaundice in the first 24 hours of life is abnormal. ● Jaundice that develops or worsens after a baby leaves the hospital should be reported to your doctor. ● Poor nursing, excessive drowsiness, irritability, and fever in a jaundiced baby should be reported immediately. ● If your infant develops jaundice follow your physician's directions to the letter.

Doctor's Treatment

Blood tests and cultures define the cause of the jaundice and its progress. To lower the bilirubin level your doctor may expose the baby to ultraviolet light or replace the infant's blood with that of a donor.

Related Topic: Jaundice In Children

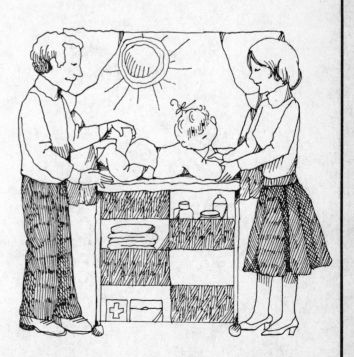

Parents should observe newborns closely in natural light in order to detect jaundice.

KNEE PAINS

Description

The knee is the most structurally complicated joint in the body. Four bones come together at the knee: the femur (thigh bone), the tibia (shin bone), the fibula (smaller, outer, lower-leg bone), and the patella (kneecap). Internally, there are two crescent-shaped cartilages and two crossed ligaments in addition to all the cartilaginous surfaces and external ligaments that are common to all joints. Because of its complexity, the knee is vulnerable and subject to a wide variety of injuries and complaints. It can be affected by rheumatoid arthritis, or injured by a puncture wound, and it can be the seat of pain without being the center of a problem; the hip might be to blame.

Active adolescents are prone to Osgood-Schlatter's disease, a painful and tender swelling of the tibial tuberosity—the bony prominence at the upper end of the shin bone, about one inch below the kneecap. When a teenager is kicking (as on a playing field) or climbing, the large muscle at the front of the thigh pulls on this tuberosity (via the kneecap) to straighten the leg. If injury cuts off blood supply to the tuberosity, it becomes swollen and tender and causes the active youth pain when the leg is straightened.

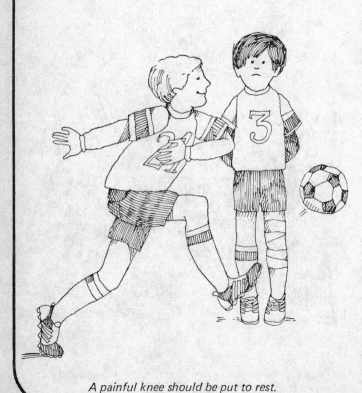

A painful knee should be put to rest.

Diagnosis

The diagnosis of the cause of knee pain depends upon the patient's history, the presence or absence of symptoms, and upon the accurate location of the pain. Tenderness at the edges of the kneecap without swelling usually indicates that the cartilage on the underside of the kneecap has been bruised and softened (chondromalacia). Swelling of the knee joint—like a fullness on both sides of the kneecap—indicates arthritis or an internal injury.

Home Treatment

Treatment depends upon the problem, but usually—as in Osgood-Schlatter's disease—it involves limiting your child's activities. For two to four weeks, or until the swelling and tenderness are gone, the knee must not be bent so that it cannot, in turn, be forcefully extended. This rules out two-legged stair climbing, bicycling, running, and jumping. An elastic knee support can be a helpful reminder during this period of healing. (Treatment of chondromalacia involves the temporary limitation of strenuous activities like track, trampoline, football, and soccer.)

Precautions

Swelling of the knee joint may be serious; it requires a doctor's attention. • If one knee cannot be straightened to match the opposite knee, fluid (blood or serum) has probably accumulated at the joint, and the knee should be seen by a doctor. • Do not put weight on a swollen knee until it has been seen by a doctor. • Remember that knee pain may mean hip trouble.

Doctor's Treatment

The doctor makes a thorough, detailed examination of each component of the knee and checks its range of normal and abnormal movement. X rays of knees and hips may be taken and, sometimes, an arthrogram (X ray after injection of radio-opaque fluid). Fluid may be drawn from the joint for diagnostic tests. Specific treatment, depending upon the diagnosis, may include bed rest, antibiotics, a cast, crutches, or surgery.

Related Topics: Arthritis, Hip Problems

Description

Laryngitis is an inflammation of the voice box (larynx). It is closely related to croup; but unlike croup, it isn't associated with breathing difficulties. Laryngitis is almost always due to a respiratory virus. Symptoms are hoarseness, dry hacking cough, scratchy throat, low-grade (101°F) or no fever. Laryngitis may last from one to fourteen days.

Diagnosis

Diagnosis is based on the typical symptoms of hoarseness and dry cough without any breathing difficulty.

Home Treatment

Plug in a vaporizer. Give your child warm drinks, and place warm compresses on his neck. Hush him gently if he tries to speak. Give him aspirin or acetaminophen for fever or pain and an expectorant cough remedy for temporary relief of cough.

Precautions

● If any breathing difficulty arises, notify a doctor. ● If a child has a climbing fever, difficulty breathing, and a cough, he may have an inflammation of the epiglottis (the structure in the back of the throat that prevents food from entering the larynx and windpipe. ● Inflammation of the epiglottis is a medical emergency; **take your child to a doctor promptly.**

Doctor's Treatment

Doctors will verify the diagnosis and rule out other conditions during the physical examination. They may take a throat culture and a complete blood count. If laryngitis is prolonged your doctor may x-ray your child's chest and neck or refer you to an ear, nose, and throat specialist.

Related Topics: Croup, Hoarseness

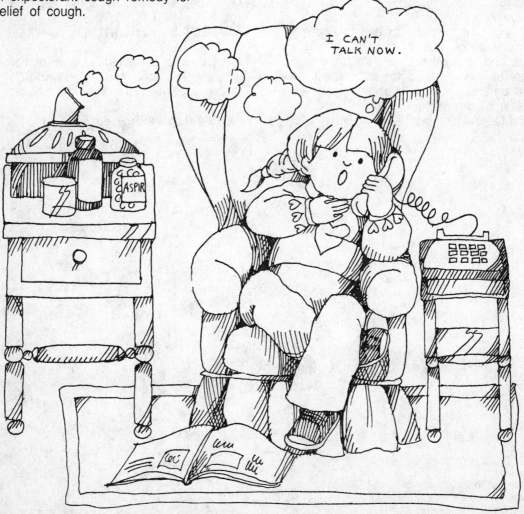

To treat laryngitis, plug in a vaporizer and have the child rest her voice.

LAZY EYE

Description

A "lazy eye" is one in which the vision is poor because a child has suppressed the image received by that eye (amblyopia ex anopsia—loss of vision from disuse). Most cases result from weakness of one or more of the six small muscles that move the eyeball. The condition also can result from marked near- or farsightedness, astigmatism, or other interference with vision in one eye (congenital cataracts, scars on the cornea, etc.)

Eye muscle weaknesses can cause the eyes to turn in or out in relation to each other. This can lead to the child's seeing double. If a young child learns to ignore one of the double images, a loss of vision in that eye results. On the other hand, if the eye muscles are normal, but the vision is poor in one eye, the young child may ignore the poor image received. This, too, can cause amblyopia and, in turn, leads to that eye turning in or out.

Diagnosis

Lazy eye should be suspected when the eyes are not parallel all or most of the time or are parallel less and less often in a child under seven years of age. Your doctor will inspect the insides and outsides of both eyes and test their movements in all directions. Vision will be checked with a letter or picture chart when your child is old enough to understand directions. A younger child's vision should be checked by an ophthalmologist using an indirect method.

Home Treatment

No home treatment is advised until a doctor has clarified the condition.

Precautions

The only precaution is catching the condition in time to correct it. See your doctor if: ● your child's eyes aren't parallel; ● the pupil of one is a different color than the other; ● your child (past the age of two) has trouble seeing or judging distances when reaching for an object; or ● your child cocks his head to one side or turns his face to see better (he may be compensating for double vision). ● Have your child's vision checked each year after age three or four. Amblyopia can be treated successfully in children up to age seven. If untreated the condition may become permanent.

Doctor's Treatment

Amblyopia is corrected by an operation, by patching the good eye or hindering the vision in the good eye with eye drops or glasses.

Related Topic: Crossed Eyes

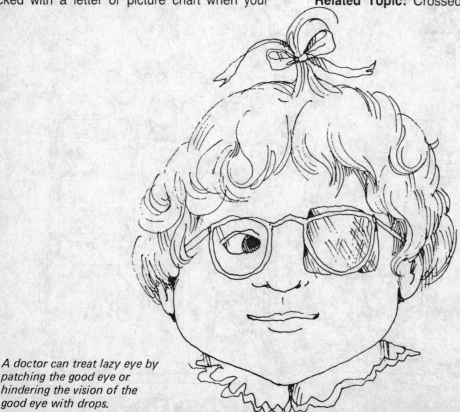

A doctor can treat lazy eye by patching the good eye or hindering the vision of the good eye with drops.

LEUKEMIA

Description

Leukemia is cancer of the white blood cells. It can afflict children at any age, but it most frequently occurs in children between three and four years old. The disease may progress slowly or rapidly. A quarter of the cases are detected during routine physical exams before the child has any symptoms.

Typical symptoms of leukemia are: anemia (indicated by paleness, weakness, or tiredness); spontaneous bruises on the body; swollen, red, and bleeding gums; low-grade fever (101°F); a visible swelling of some lymph nodes (not tender and not red); bone pain; uncontrollable and frequently recurrent nosebleeds; and blood in the urine or stools.

Diagnosis

Doctors may suspect the disease when a physical exam reveals the above signs and symptoms and an enlarged spleen or liver. Suspicion is strengthened by an abnormal blood count that shows malignant white blood cells. The diagnosis is confirmed by an examination of bone marrow.

Home Treatment

None.

Precautions

Although it is rare, leukemia is one of the four "common" forms of cancer in children. Many illnesses imitate leukemia, and they are NOT rare; for example, infectious mononucleosis, herpes infections of the mouth, vitamin C deficiency, rheumatic fever, rheumatoid arthritis, sickle cell anemia, and other diseases that cause spontaneous bruising. Do not jump to the conclusion that your child has leukemia because of the presence of any of the above signs or symptoms. See your doctor to ease your mind.

Doctor's Treatment

Today, leukemia can be treated with a wide range of anticancer drugs. These drugs may result in long periods of remission and perhaps even cure. Pediatric oncologists (cancer specialists) choose and supervise the treatment of leukemia.

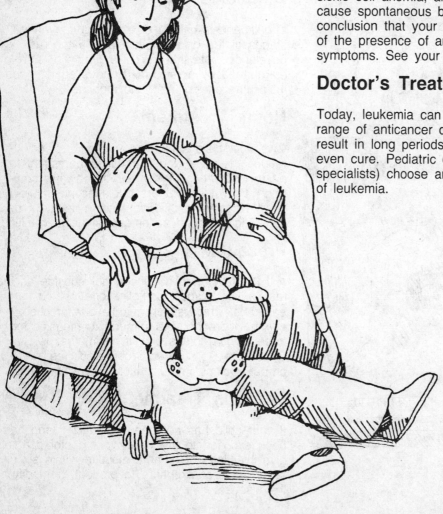

Leukemia can be successfully treated with a wide variety of drugs prescribed by a doctor.

MEASLES

Description

Also known as *rubeola*, measles is a highly contagious illness caused by a specific virus. It is characterized by a high fever, severe cough, and a rash, and frequently sparks severe complications. Measles passes from child to child by an airborne or droplet-borne virus; it has an incubation period of ten to twelve days. The disease can be passed on to others any time between the fifth day of incubation period through the first few days of the rash.

Measles' first symptoms are a runny nose, reddish eyes, cough, and fever. After three or four days the fever rises to 104°F or 105°F, the cough worsens and a heavy, splotchy, red rash begins on the neck and face. The rash quickly spreads over the trunk, arms, and legs. When the rash has erupted fully, the fever breaks, and the child improves if no complications set in.

Common complications of a bout with measles include viral and bacterial pneumonias and middle ear infections. Encephalitis (inflammation of the brain) occurs in one or two of every 1,000 cases.

Measles in children who have received only the dead virus vaccine produces a high fever, prostration, and a rash of blisters and petechiae (purplish-red spots). It often is complicated by pneumonia.

Diagnosis

The diagnosis cannot be made during early stages of the disease. Just before the rash develops, spots that look like grains of salt surrounded by a red rim (Koplik's spots) appear inside the cheeks near the molars.

Home Treatment

Give your child aspirin or acetaminophen to reduce the fever and a cough suppressant to ease a severe cough. Keep him away from bright light; light bothers but does not injure the eyes. Have your child drink extra liquids if he can, and give him antiemetics if he is vomiting.

Precautions

• If the fever and cough do not subside as the rash peaks suspect complications. Watch for earaches, which signify middle ear infection.
• A newborn baby is immune to measles for three to six months only if his mother is immune. • Be sure your child receives the proper, lifelong immunization against measles.

Doctor's Treatment

If your child has not been immunized and has been exposed to the virus, your doctor can give injections of gamma globulin within six or seven days of exposure to prevent or modify the disease.

Injections of gamma globulin will prevent or modify measles if an unimmunized child has been exposed.

Related Topics: Earaches, Encephalitis, Immunizations, Pneumonia

MENINGITIS

Description

Meningitis is an infection of the meninges, the layers of tissue that cover and protect the brain and spinal cord. Most often, meningitis is caused by infection by one of three bacteria: meningococcus, pneumococcus, or hemophilus influenzae. Usually contracted by direct contact with, or airborn droplets, from a healthy carrier, meningitis seldom is spread by a person with the disease. Its incubation period is one to seven days.

Meningitis may be a complication of a skull fracture if the fracture has extended into the nose, middle ear, or nasal sinus. Sometimes, meningitis follows an upper respiratory tract infection or middle ear infection. Its characteristic symptoms are moderate to high fever, headache, vomiting, prostration, convulsions, and a stiff neck—the child cannot touch his chin to his chest with his mouth closed. The tripod sign in which the child sits with his arms braced behind him for support is typical. (Purplish red spots called petechiae scattered over the body together with fever indicate a probable meningococcus infection.)

Diagnosis

The diagnosis only can be made with certainty by testing spinal fluid obtained by a spinal tap.

Home Treatment

Meningitis is a medical emergency in which hours, if not minutes, count. **Do not attempt any home treatment.**

Precautions

The unnecessary use of antibiotics for an upper respiratory tract infection may mask the onset of meningitis. A child who is prostrated with fever and a stiff neck and has petechiae on the body is in danger and should be taken to a medical facility immediately.

Doctor's Treatment

Your doctor will take a complete history and perform a physical and neurologic exam, followed by a spinal tap. Spinal fluid will be examined for cells, bacteria, and abnormal chemical components. (This is the only way to differentiate between meningitis and encephalitis, which is also a life-threatening disease.) A culture of the spinal fluid, blood, nose and throat mucus, and petechiae may also be done. Immediately following the spinal tap and cultures your doctor will administer intravenous fluids and antibiotics and possibly prescribe two antibiotics if the infecting organism is unknown. If your child has been exposed to meningococcal meningitis or to hemophilus influenzae, your doctor may choose to administer penicillin, sulfonamide, or rifampin. Vaccines against meningococci, pneumococci, and hemophilus influenzae are available, but they are not currently recommended for general use.

Related Topics: Earaches, Encephalitis, Fractures

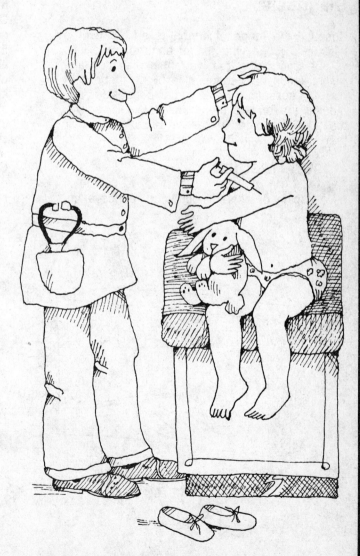

If your child has been exposed to meningitis, your doctor may choose to administer penicillin, sulfonamide, or rifampin.

125

MENSTRUATION

Description

Girls in the United States begin to menstruate somewhere between nine and seventeen years of age. The average age is 12. Following the onset of menstruation (menarche), it may take from several months to five years for the hormones to balance and produce regular menstrual periods. During this time, no menstrual irregularity is necessarily abnormal.

For about five percent of adolescent girls abdominal cramps and backaches—which last one or two days at the start of a menstrual period—may be severe enough to interfere with normal activities. In many instances cramps and backaches are related to emotional factors such as tension or anxiety. They also may be due to a hormonal imbalance or pelvic disease.

Diagnosis

Because the range of normal is so broad, it is difficult to judge whether an abnormality exists or not. Symptoms that warrant explanation are menstruation before age nine or no menses by age 17; cessation of menstrual periods for six months (or for one month in a sexually active teenager); repeated excessive bleeding; or pain that inteferes with normal activity.

Home Treatment

Give aspirin or acetaminophen to reduce any

mild, transient pain. Encourage your daughter to maintain her normal activities during her menstrual period.

Precautions

● The facts about menstruation should be explained to your preteen daughter to correct any "old wive's tales" she may have heard from others and to prepare her for this event of maturation. Many good books are on the market for parents and teenagers which may alleviate any embarrassment and correct any misinformation.

Doctor's Treatment

If problems arise your doctor should conduct a complete physical examination, which includes a rectal and a limited pelvic examination. Chromosome studies and evaluation of the girls' hormonal status may also be conducted. Sometimes tests of the thyroid gland activity and other blood tests will be ordered. Rarely will a dilatation and curettage (D & C) or laparoscopy examination of the interior of the abdomen be necessary. A pregnancy test may be called for under the appropriate circumstances. Your doctor may well find no abnormality and no treatment will be necessary. Oral cyclic hormones may be prescribed for two or three periods or an iron supplement or thyroid medication if indicated.

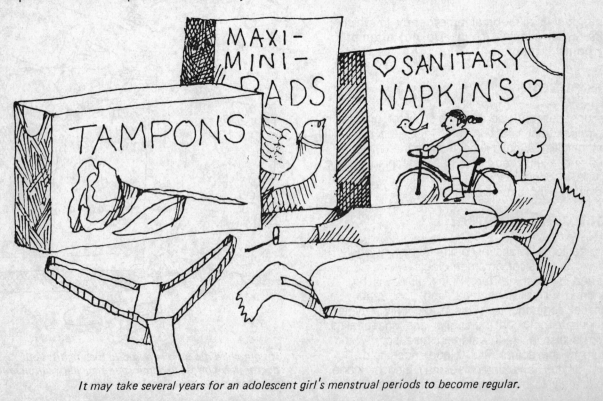

It may take several years for an adolescent girl's menstrual periods to become regular.

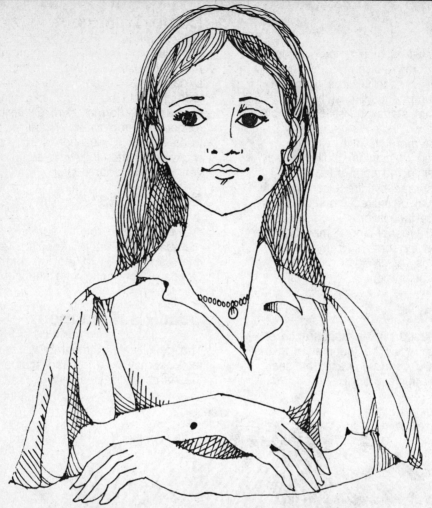

Moles may be considered beauty marks; most are harmless.

Description

Moles are benign tumors of the skin. They may be flat, dome-shaped, or protruding. They vary in color from tan or brown to blue or black and in size from one-sixteenth to one-half inch or larger. Rarely, if ever, are moles present at birth; they develop sporadically during childhood. No child is totally free of moles, and some develop hundreds of them.

   The possibility of any mole becoming malignant (cancerous) is remote. An exception is a mole called the *extensive pigmented nevus.* This mole is extremely large (several inches wide) and dark, is present at birth, and may become malignant.

Diagnosis

The diagnosis generally is based on inspection of the mole. Microscopic examination of an entire mole may be needed for some doubtful skin tumors.

Home Treatment

None.

Precautions

Moles should be seen by a doctor if: • they have been partly removed by accident; • they are bleeding or crusting; • they are changing color or growing rapidly; • or if their pigment is moving into the surrounding skin.

Doctor's Treatment

Your doctor will surgically remove any moles if the above conditions are evident. A mole may also be removed for cosmetic reasons. (All extensive pigmented nevuses probably should be surgically removed because of the possibility of a malignancy.) Moles must be removed completely by excising them with a scalpel. The surgery will leave a scar of some sort. They cannot safely be burned off by an electrocautery, acids, dry ice, or liquid nitrogen.

MOLLUSCUM CONTAGIOSUM

Description

Often mistaken for warts or pimples, molluscum contagiosum is a common, chronic infection of the skin caused by a specific virus. Each molluscum is a plump, round, slightly waxy looking "pimple" that starts one-sixteenth inch in size and slowly grows to a diameter of one-quarter inch or more. It is firm to the touch. In the course of months, mollusca may spread and number in the hundreds.

The disease is spread by direct contact with an infected individual or indirect contact with personal articles. Its incubation period is long—two to seven weeks—and it may become secondarily infected by scratching. Molluscum contagiosum spreads rapidly through other rashes but carries no systemic symptoms.

Diagnosis

The diagnosis is based on the appearance of the pimple-like eruptions. The indentation in the center of each molluscum can easily be seen on close inspection in good light.

Home Treatment

If mollusca are few in number they may respond to applications of tincture of iodine twice a day. To apply the iodine use a toothpick and be careful to avoid touching surrounding, normal skin. Occasionally, mollusca respond to applications of terramycin ointment twice a day. If mollusca do not disappear in two weeks after following either treatment take your child to your doctor.

Precautions

● The condition readily spreads among members of a family; keep the soiled clothing, linen, and towels of the infected child separate. Ordinary laundering with soap or detergent kills the virus.

Doctor's Treatment

The definitive treatment is to incise each molluscum with a pointed scalpel and remove the hard, white, pearl-like center.

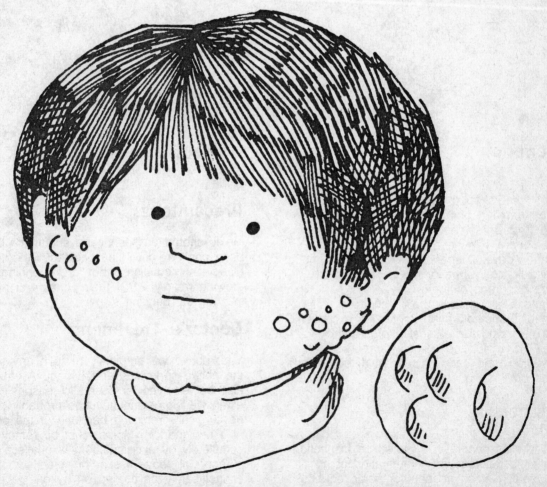

Molluscum contagiosum has only one symptom--a characteristic rash.

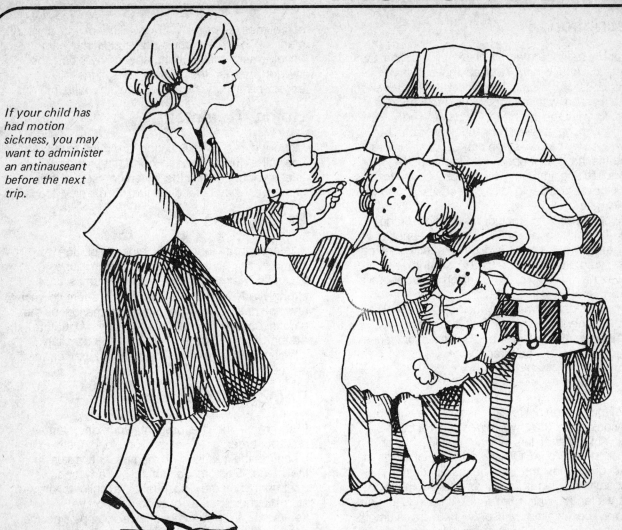

If your child has had motion sickness, you may want to administer an antinauseant before the next trip.

Description

Car, air, and sea sickness are all forms of motion sickness. Sufficient rhythmic motion up and down or side to side will make most children nauseated, presumably because of the effect on the balance mechanism of the inner ears. Some children are more susceptible than others; young infants are apparently immune.

A motion-sick child becomes nauseated, pale or "green," and anxious; he may perspire and vomit. Motion sickness is not self-induced nor can the victim control it. It can be serious.

Diagnosis

Motion sickness is fairly obvious. Susceptible children will have recurrent attacks.

Home Treatment

Consult your doctor about antinauseants. Give your child an antinauseant by mouth one hour before the start of each trip and every four hours during the trip. Dimenhydrinate antinauseant tablets or liquid are highly effective and safe. The antinauseants and promethazine, meclizine, and chlorpromazine are also effective. Prochlorperazine antiemetic is not recommended for children. Lying down with eyes closed, coolness, preoccupation with a game, and a light diet will minimize motion sickness.

Precautions

● Prolonged motion sickness (over hours) can eventually result in excessive vomiting, vomiting of blood, and dehydration.

Doctor's Treatment

Your doctor's treatment will be the same as your home treatment unless your child's symptoms have progressed to dehydration and gastric bleeding, which require hospitalization and intravenous fluids.

Related Topics: Dehydration, Vomiting

MUMPS

Description

Mumps is a moderately contagious infection by a specific virus which involves the salivary glands. It is contracted by contact with saliva from a person with mumps. The incubation period for mumps is 14 to 21 days. The disease can be passed on any time from two or more days before symptoms appear until all symptoms have disappeared. One attack confers lifelong immunity; if attacks seem to recur, they are due to other diseases of the salivary gland.

Typical symptoms include fever (low-grade 101°F or as high as 105°F), loss of appetite, and headache. One or two days after onset of these symptoms, one or more salivary glands become painfully swollen; swelling lasts about a week.

Complications of mumps include encephalitis and permanent deafness. The disease may even involve the ovaries and testicles or cause an infection of the pancreas.

Diagnosis

The diagnosis of a typical case of the mumps is obvious from the swelling of the parotid salivary gland that lies behind, below, and in front of the earlobe. Only a swelling of the parotid gland has the earlobe as its center. Other salivary glands, such as the submaxillary salivary glands, which lie under the edge of the jaw, may be swollen with or without involvement of the parotids, and swelling may occur on one or both sides of the face.

Problems of diagnosis arise when complications of mumps develop before, or sometimes even without, swelling of the salivary glands. Then, the cause of abdominal pain (involvement of the pancreas or ovaries), the swollen, tender testicles, or the signs of encephalitis may be difficult to link with mumps.

Home Treatment

Moderate rest and isolation are recommended until all symptoms have gone. Aspirin or acetaminophen may be given to reduce pain and fever. Avoid feeding the child spicy foods.

Precautions

● Infants from four to six months of age are immune only if their mothers are immune.
● Routine immunization against mumps is strongly advised. ● Attacks which seem to recur are not due to mumps but inflammation of the parotid salivary gland (often allergic in nature), a stone in the salivary duct, or a bacterial infection of the gland. They should be reported to your doctor.

Doctor's Treatment

If complications are present, your doctor may have to order a spinal tap or blood tests to measure the number of mumps antibodies in the blood. Doctors do not follow any specific treatment, but may hospitalize a child to arrive at a diagnosis or to provide supportive treatment. A child may receive mumps vaccine shortly after exposure to the disease.

Related Topics: Encephalitis, Immunizations

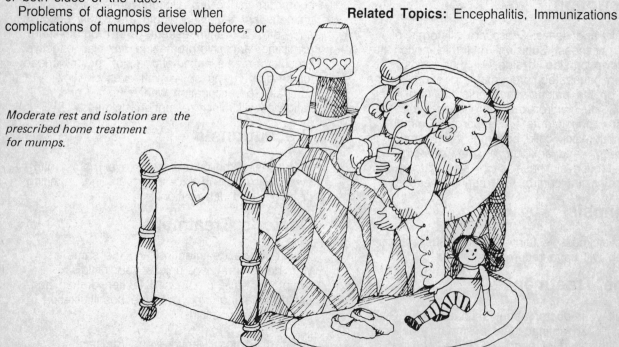

Moderate rest and isolation are the prescribed home treatment for mumps.

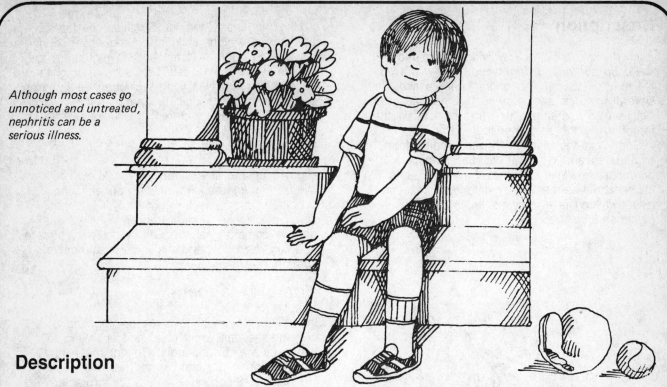

Although most cases go unnoticed and untreated, nephritis can be a serious illness.

Description

The most common form of nephritis in children is an inflammation of the kidneys that follows such streptococcal infections as strep throat, scarlet fever and streptococcal impetigo. One attack usually confers lifelong immunity.

The first symptoms of nephritis develop one to three weeks after the onset of a strep infection. They are usually mild. Urine may be smoky, brownish-red with blood, or scant and urination infrequent. The eyes of an infected child may become puffy. Fever (101°F to 104°F) may be present for several days.

Occasionally, nephritis starts abruptly, and the illness is severe. At these times it produces high fever and excessive blood in the urine followed by: complete or almost complete cessation of urination; headache; vomiting; high blood pressure; and convulsions.

Most children recover completely. Urination generally returns to normal in a matter of weeks. A few develop chronic kidney disease, however.

Diagnosis

A urinalysis report can confirm the disease. Often streptococcal organisms can be cultured from the nose and throat, also supporting diagnosis.

Home Treatment

Most cases of nephritis probably go unnoticed, undiagnosed and pass without treatment. If the symptoms are recognized nephritis is serious enough for your child to see the doctor. No home treatment is recommended.

Precautions

Be suspicious of ● the possibility of nephritis following a sore throat whether or not the sore throat has been treated with antibiotics, ● scanty, dark urine; ● and puffiness around the eyes.

Doctor's Treatment

Your doctor will perform a complete physical check-up, measuring the blood pressure, carrying out a neurologic examination, and looking at the eye grounds. A urinalysis, blood test, and perhaps a throat culture can further identify a streptococcal infection. If nephritis is found, your doctor will treat the condition with penicillin for ten days; a severe case of nephritis may require hospitalization for observation, reduction of high blood pressure, and treatment of convulsions.

Your doctor will monitor your child's urine and blood until they return to normal. Bed rest is recommended only during the acute phase of the disease. Oral penicillin may be prescribed for several months, both while the child is recovering and afterward.

Related Topics: Convulsions with Fever, Headaches, Impetigo, Strep Throat, Vomiting

NIGHTMARES

Description

A child experiencing a terrifying dream may wake up screaming, frightened, and wild-eyed. He may be disoriented or frantically active for several minutes and may or may not recall the details of the dream. Often the incident will be forgotten by the next morning.

Some experts distinguish bad dreams from nightmares and night terrors. For practical purposes, however, all three have the same cause and treatment; they differ only in degree. (Sleepwalking is also a manifestation of nightmares.)

In a nightmare, the mind relives the fears and anxieties your child has experienced during his waking hours. Occasionally a nightmare may be the result of the usual stresses your child encounters in his daily life. Frequent nightmares are abnormal and indicate unreasonable pressures on the child.

Diagnosis

High fever and illness have been known to induce nightmares. When this happens, the condition resembles delirium and should pass when the illness is cleared-up. (Measles was once a common cause.) Otherwise, a nightmare is easily identified and the initial treatment of comfort given.

Home Treatment

Immediate treatment involves holding and hugging the distraught child and speaking to him calmly and soothingly. Do not make any effort to rouse the child to full consciousness too quickly. Sleepwalkers must be protected from falls or other injuries.

The basic home treatment is to seek out and relieve the sources of undue stress. Most nightmares are the result of: school problems (fear of failure or teacher-student conflicts); peer problems (playing with older children, being bullied, sexual experimentation); and intrafamily pressures (marital friction, alcoholism, physical or emotional abuse, divorce, hospitalization, death). Prohibition or strict monitoring of television viewing may relieve another cause. Not only monsters and violence but newscasts and cartoons can arouse anxieties in children.

Doctor's Treatment

Your doctor may recommend the temporary use of sedatives or tranquilizers to relieve nightmares. But for a long-range cure, your doctor will try to uncover the cause of your child's anxieties through investigation of his daily relationships and experiences. Assistance from school psychiatric personnel may be sought.

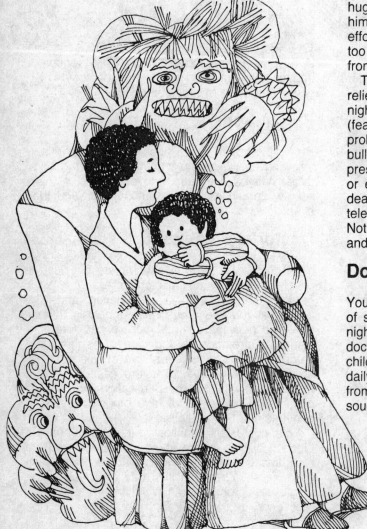

Reassure a child woken up by a nightmare.

Description

Nosebleeds are as much a part of normal childhood as scraped knees and bruised shins. Ninety-nine percent of them arise from the rupture of tiny blood vessels in the septum (midline partition of the nose) located about one-quarter inch in from the nostrils. These small arteries, veins, and capillaries are easily broken by a minor blow to the nose. A scab forms during healing and is easily disturbed by rubbing or picking, which reactivates the bleeding. This sequence of events may be further aggravated by: allergies or a head cold that dilate the blood vessels in the nose; heated air that dries out the nasal membranes; sneezing, coughing, and blowing the nose; and by a child rubbing and scratching his nose, especially during sleep (most nosebleeds start at night).

Diagnosis

A nosebleed is fairly obvious. Since the two sides of the nose join in the back and with the throat and the esophagus (which lead to the stomach), blood may flow from both nostrils, from the mouth, and may be vomited.

Home Treatment

Your child should be taught at an early age how to stop a nosebleed by himself. He should be instructed to remain calm and to sit upright with his head held high to decrease blood pressure. He should grasp the whole lower half of his nose between his thumb and fingers and compress both sides in this way firmly against the septum. The nose should be held for ten minutes to allow the blood to clot. If bleeding recurs when the pressure is released, a large clot in the nose probably is preventing the broken blood vessel from retracting. Have your child blow his nose vigorously to dislodge the clot. After the clot has been removed, repeat compression of the nose for ten to twelve minutes.

To prevent recurring nosebleeds, put ointment (petroleum jelly or antibiotic ointment) up the nose in the morning and evening for seven to fourteen days. Add moisture to the night air with a vaporizer or humidifier. Give the child antihistamines if he has an allergy or oral decongestants if he has a head cold.

Precautions

● Do not merely pinch nostrils together but compress the entire soft portion of the nose. Otherwise, the blood simply will dam up and run down the throat. ● Do not lay your child down. ● Remain calm and reassure your child. ● Cold compresses, pressure on the upper lip, nose drops, and other household remedies are unnecessary. ● Do not pack the nose with cotton or gauze.

Doctor's Treatment

Generally, your doctor's treatment will be the same as your home treatment and is necessary only when you are unable to follow the above directions. If the nosebleed is due to an allergy or a cold your doctor will treat those conditions. Your doctor will rarely need to use cocaine or epinephrine, pack the passage, or treat a recurring nosebleed by cauterizing the nose. An ointment containing estrogens may be recommended to prevent recurrences of a nosebleed.

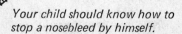

Your child should know how to stop a nosebleed by himself.

PERLECHE

Description

Cracks or fissures at the edges of the mouth that become red, sore, and crusted are called perleche. These cracks may bleed when the mouth is opened wide. Classically, perleche is a sign of a vitamin B deficiency, common in India but almost unknown in the United States. Of those cases that occur in this country almost all are caused by an irritation from toothpastes. Chemicals in mouthwashes, orthodontic or dental materials, or from plastic toys also cause the condition.

Diagnosis

Chronic, painful sores where upper and lower lips meet are the telling signs of perleche. Occasionally, perleche may be confused with or occur along with fever blisters or impetigo.

Home Treatment

Stop the use of your normal toothpaste temporarily, and have your child brush his teeth with table salt or bicarbonate of soda. After perleche heals, try other toothpastes or ask your dentist for advice.

Precautions

• If the condition does not clear up after the child has stopped using toothpaste, mouthwashes, or other oral chemicals, take him to a dentist or doctor.

Doctor's Treatment

Your doctor's treatment is the same as the suggested home treatment, although your doctor also may need to concentrate on treating a secondary staphylococcal or streptococcal infection. Although steroid ointments tend to hasten healing, they can confuse the doctor's efforts to find the cause of the condition. Comparable medications will be provided.

Related Topics: Herpes Simplex, Impetigo

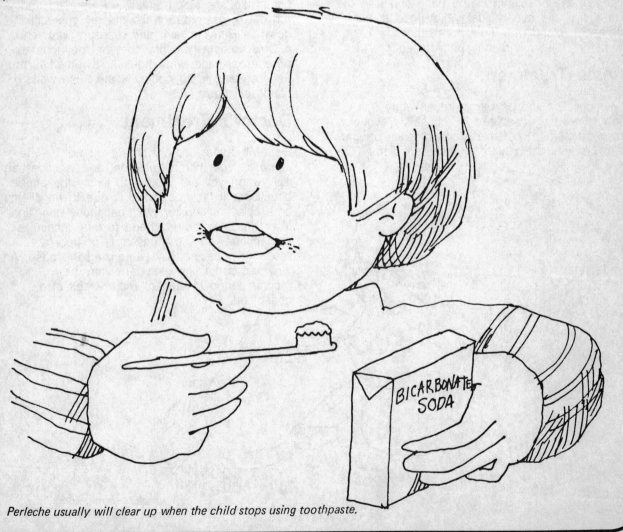

Perleche usually will clear up when the child stops using toothpaste.

Description

Toeing-in of the feet, particularly when standing and walking, is known as pigeon toes. After birth, the position and shape of the feet and legs reflect the position they held during the last weeks *in utero*. By the age of three months, the child's feet and legs should have assumed a normal shape.

Throughout infancy and early childhood, the position of the feet and legs can be influenced by the manner in which they are held while the child is lying down and sitting. If the child habitually sleeps face down with his toes directed inward, pigeon toes development is encouraged. Sitting on the haunches with the knees sharply flexed and the toes directed outward also may lead to pigeon toes.

Pigeon toes also may result from a deformity of the foot (*adductovarus deformity*), the lower leg (*tibial torsion*), or the thigh bone (*femoral torsion or femoral anteversion*). Depending on the severity of the deformity, the child's toes will point inward to a great or small degree. A child who has a marked deformity will tend to trip over his feet until he learns to compensate for the handicap.

Diagnosis

An *adductovarus deformity* of the foot can be determined by laying a straight edge along the outer border of the child's foot. If the outer border of the foot is not absolutely straight from the heel to the little toe, the child has adductovarus deformity. To discern *tibial torsion* place the infant or child on his back with his legs straight out, kneecaps pointed upward, and ankles at right angles to the lower leg. If the toes do not point straight up but toward the midline, the child has tibial torsion.

Femoral torsion or *anteversion* usually does not begin until age four or five and from then on gradually worsens. It can be detected by rotating the thighs at the hip joint. If the thighs make a larger arc internally than externally the child has femoral torsion.

Home Treatment

By three months of age, your infant will prefer to sleep with his toes directed outward. This position is normal and should be encouraged. When your child is old enough to sit upright, his feet should be straight or turned outward. And until eighteen to twenty-four months, your toddler usually will walk with one or both feet turned outward for a wider base and better balance. This, too, is normal. A tendency to toe in after three months of age should be called to your doctor's attention.

Precautions

● An uncorrected adductovarus deformity makes proper shoe-fitting difficult and eventually may lead to a skewed foot with bunions in adolescence or adulthood. A child who sits on the floor should be taught to sit cross-legged, not on his haunches with his toes directed outward. ● Corrective orthopedic shoes should be prescribed only by a medical professional, not by a shoe salesman. ● Most minor cases of pigeon toes correct themselves. Nevertheless, let a doctor help you judge whether the condition is minor or not.

Doctor's Treatment

Your doctor will observe your child while he stands and walks with and without shoes. The feet, lower and upper legs, and the rotation of the hips will be examined. If a case of pigeon toes is mild, nothing need be done. To correct adductovarus deformity after three months of age, your doctor will order specific kinds of shoes or plaster casts. To correct tibial torsion, a splint that holds the feet outwardly rotated while the child sleeps will be prescribed. Your doctor will probably not treat femoral anteversion until your child is an adolescent. If the condition has not corrected itself by that time, surgery on the thigh bones may be necessary.

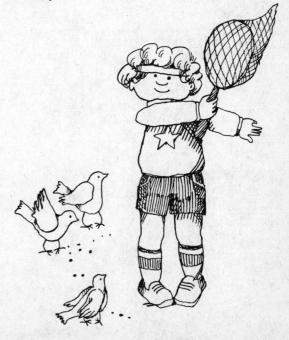

Most minor cases of pigeon toes will correct themselves.

PINWORMS

Description

The pinworm, a distant cousin of the earthworm, lives only in humans and the higher apes. The adult pinworm is one-quarter to one-half inch in length, white in color, and about as thick as stout, sewing thread. It lives in the large intestine and, moving with a caterpillar-like motion, comes out at night to lay its microscopic-size eggs on the skin around the anus. The eggs are transmitted from the skin to the mouth by the hands or via toys and food and are swallowed. The eggs hatch, and two to six weeks later the larvae have developed into mature, egg-laying adult pinworms and the cycle continues. (Pinworms may be transmitted to other children and to adults in the same manner described above.)

A child with pinworms will have few symptoms. He may complain at night of itching or burning around the anal or genital area. If the infestation is heavy he may have abdominal cramps. Pinworms may cause appendicitis (though rarely), and they may work their way into a girl's vagina and urethra causing vaginitis and cystitis to develop.

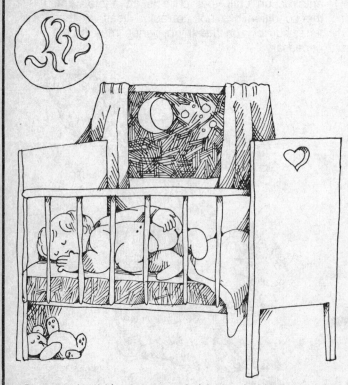

Pinworms could be the cause of nighttime itchiness around the anal area.

Diagnosis

Usually the diagnosis is easily made by examining the skin around the anus at night while the child sleeps or just after he has awakened. Pinworms head back into the anus if disturbed by light; so the search must be done quickly. A pinworm can be mistaken for lint on the skin; if the lint moves, it is a pinworm. Occasionally, pinworms may be found in a bowel movement, but this is not reliable.

Home Treatment

Vermifuges (worm medicines) must be obtained by prescription, but many doctors will prescribe them over the telephone. One vermifuge—mebendazole—is available in chewable tablets; the dosage is one tablet regardless of weight. Another medication—pyrvinium pamoate is given in amounts equaling one teaspoon or one tablet for every 22 pounds of weight up to a maximum of seven tablets or teaspoons per day. One teaspoon or one tablet of piperazine citrate is given for every 15 pounds of weight for seven days (up to a maximum of seven tablets or teaspoons per daily dose). Twice a day, 12.5 mg of thiabendazole may be given for every pound of weight; or once a day, one teaspoon of pyrantel pamoate may be given for every ten pounds of weight up to a maximum of four teaspoons. The course of treatment with any of these drugs may be repeated once or twice if you allow seven to ten days between each series. When one member of a family has pinworms, all members (except infants) should receive treatment.

Precautions

● Suspect that pinworms may be the cause of recurrent cystitis or vaginitis. ● If one member of a family has pinworms, launder his underclothes, bed linens, and towels to destroy the worms' eggs. Also, cut and scrub his fingernails to remove any eggs. ● Do not mistake lint or thread for pinworms; look for movement. ● Do not blame household cats and dogs for pinworms. These worms live only in humans.

Doctor's Treatment

Your doctor will investigate for pinworms using a National Institutes of Health swab or tape with which eggs from the skin can be picked up. A microscopic examination will be made of the swab or tape. The doctor's treatment will be the same as your home treatment.

PITYRIASIS ROSEA

Description

Pityriasis rosea is a common, harmless, long-lasting disease which goes unrecognized by most parents. Generally, it affects teenagers and young adults, but it may occur at any age. The disease is almost certainly caused by a virus, but the specific germ has not been discovered. It is mildly contagious, but isolation is not considered necessary. One attack confers lifelong immunity.

In most cases of pityriasis rosea the first sign is a single patch (herald patch) the size of a nickel or quarter on the skin of the trunk or extremities. Round or oval, the patch is salmon-colored (pink or reddish) and slightly crinkled in the center; it is slightly scaly at the edge. The patch is not tender but may itch. Occasionally it is accompanied by headache, lethargy, pain in the joints, and a sore throat. Five to fourteen days after the appearance of the herald patch, 10 to 100 spots break out on the body; each is similar in appearance to, but smaller than, the original patch. The rash does not affect the face, forearms, and lower legs of an older child, but it may not spare these areas in younger children. The rash lasts for three to eight weeks, during which time the child feels fine.

Diagnosis

The diagnosis is based on the characteristic

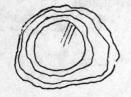

appearance of the rash. Some of the spots are round, but others are oval. The identifiable feature of the oval spots is the long axis that is parallel to the lines of skin cleavage. Spots on the chest, back, and abdomen have a long axis that is parallel to the ribs, for example.

Home Treatment

No treatment is necessary. Itching, if present, can be relieved by administering oral antihistamines. Bathing with a soft soap and exposure to sunlight apparently shorten the duration of the rash.

Precautions

- The appearance of the herald patch may suggest ringworm, eczema, or impetigo; but when the patch does not respond to treatment for any of these conditions, consider pityriasis.
- The sudden blossoming of secondary spots may suggest the presence of ringworm; but ringworm does not spread in a matter of a few days.

Doctor's Treatment

None is required. However, your doctor may recommend the use of steroid ointments, oral steroids, or ultraviolet light.

Related Topics: Eczema, Impetigo, Ringworm

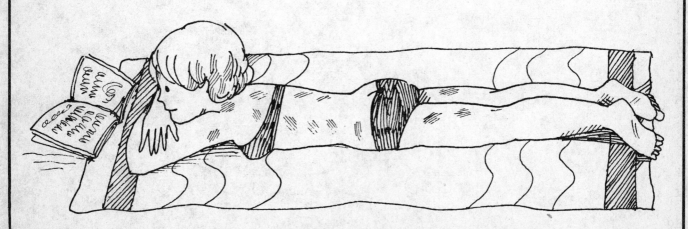

Exposure to sunlight may alleviate the rash of pityriasis rosea.

PNEUMONIA

Description

Pneumonia is an infection of one or more areas of the lungs that is caused by bacteria or a virus. The common bacterial cause of pneumonia is pneumococcus; less often, it is streptococcus or staphylococcus. The viral causes include the influenza and parainfluenza viruses, the respiratory syncytial virus, and adenoviruses. Pneumonia also may be caused by mycoplasma organisms.

Bacterial pneumonia. To contract bacterial pneumonia requires the simultaneous presence of a causative germ and a receptive host. Pneumococci, streptococci, and staphylococci frequently are present in the nose and throat of healthy children. Before these organisms can invade the lungs, however, your child's resistance must be lowered by a cold or some other upper respiratory tract infection. So bacterial pneumonia is not considered to be contagious in the usual sense.

The symptoms of bacterial pneumonia include a mild upper respiratory tract infection, followed by the sudden onset of high fever (105°F), chills, cough, rapid breathing, and sometimes pain on either or both sides of the chest. In infants the respiratory distress may cause flaring of the nostrils, retractions of the soft spaces of the chest, and grunting sounds on exhalation.

Viral pneumonia. These so-called walking pneumonias are contagious. The incubation period for mycoplasma is one to three weeks, for most viruses two to five days. The onset of viral pneumonia is gradual, creating symptoms of headache, fatigue, fever of variable (100°F-105°F) degrees, a sore throat, and a severe, dry cough.

Diagnosis

The diagnosis requires careful examination of the chest, X rays, a complete blood count, and cultures of the blood and the sputum.

Home Treatment

Many cases of viral pneumonia, mild and unrecognized, treated with cold remedies, subside spontaneously after ten to fourteen days.

Precautions

● Sudden worsening of a cold coupled with high fever, cough, chills, chest pain, or rapid breathing suggests pneumonia. ● In infants flaring of the nostrils, retractions of the chest, and grunting breathing are serious symptoms and warrant immediate medical care. ● In children sputum tinged with blood may or may not be serious, but it indicates the need for a doctor's attention.

Doctor's Treatment

Your doctor will diagnose pneumonia by means of the physical examination and laboratory tests. In the past a child with pneumonia was always hospitalized. Now, only the youngest and the most severely ill are hospitalized.

Most pneumonias respond to antibiotics. A patient with pneumococcal pneumonia will rally rapidly once antibiotics are begun. Another, with a streptococcal or staphylococcal infection, may require in-hospital administration of the antibiotics. Mycoplasma pneumonia responds to some antibiotics, but viral pneumonias do not.

Related Topic: Common Cold

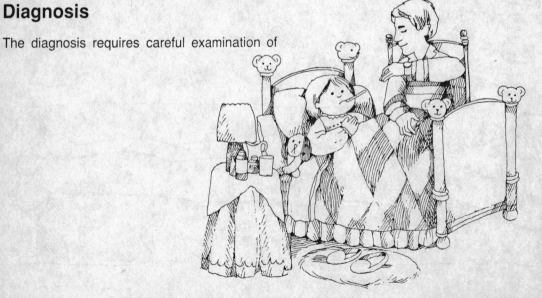

Many cases of viral pneumonia go unrecognized and are treated with cold remedies.

Description

Rashes among children in the two to twelve year age group are generally due to contact with certain agents, the most common of which is vine poison ivy. (Other weeds, such as poison oak and poison sumac, and toys, cosmetics, and chemicals used in the manufacture of clothing and shoes are also responsible.)

Poison ivy rash develops in sensitive children after direct contact with any part of the vine. It also may occur after exposure to smoke from the burning vine or from the coats of pets that have rolled in the plant. Poison ivy rash can be spread to any part of the skin by the hands, fingernails, and contaminated clothing.

Itching develops within two to twenty-four hours after contact with poison ivy. It is followed by a reddening and swelling (edema) of the skin. Pin-sized, clear blisters develop and may merge to create blisters as large as one-half inch. The rash often appears in straight lines where the plant has brushed against the skin or where the child has scratched. Poison ivy is often carried to a boy's penis by his hands.

Diagnosis

A blistered, itching rash that appears in straight lines is indicative of poison ivy. However, the rash may appear generally over the skin and look similar to other rashes.

Home Treatment

Promptly bathing the child with soap and water and cutting and scrubbing the fingernails will remove much of the poison ivy from the skin. Laundering removes it from contaminated clothing.

The most effective treatment of a small rash is to rub in a steroid ointment three or four times a day. Large rashes are best treated by oral steroids for four to five days. Check with your doctor. Calamine lotion and oral antihistamines lessen the itching.

Precautions

• If poison ivy continues to spread after four to seven days, your child is still coming into contact with the plant, directly or indirectly. Try to find the source. • Scratching can result in impetigo; so watch for signs of infection.
• Teach your child to recognize the vine.
• Make sure your child is dressed appropriately (in long pants and socks) when in the woods or around campsites.

Doctor's Treatment

Your doctor will confirm the diagnosis, treat any secondary infection, and prescribe steroids as needed. Vaccines designed to desensitize people against poison ivy are available, but they are not always effective. Oral preparations are even less helpful.

Related Topic: Impetigo

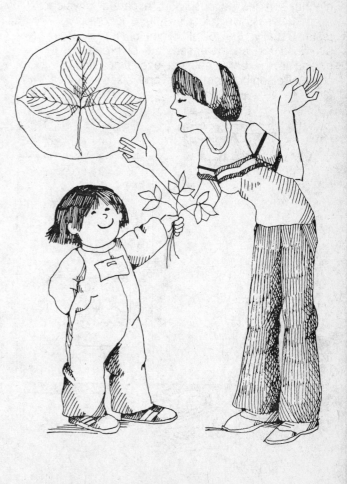

Teach your child to recognize poison ivy.

POISONING

Description

If ingested in a large enough quantity any substance, even water, can be poisonous. But some substances are more apt to be swallowed in injurious amounts, either accidentally or deliberately, than others. In the United States the usual cause of poisoning among children between the ages of one and five years is an overdose of aspirin. Then come soaps, detergents, cleansers, bleaches, vitamins, iron tonics, insecticides, plants, polishes and waxes, hormones, and tranquilizers. Less common but more toxic poisons include boric acid, oil of wintergreen, volatile hydrocarbons (gasoline, kerosine, turpentine, naphtha, cleaning fluids), strong acids, alkalis (drain and oven cleaners), and many prescription and over-the-counter medications (including aspirin substitutes and acetaminophens).

Diagnosis

The diagnosis of poisoning depends primarily upon an accurate history. Without one, the diagnosis relies on suspicion, a careful physical examination for telltale clues, and laboratory tests. Usually, the telltale signs of aspirin overdose are an increased rate of breathing, ringing in the ears, nausea, excitation, and coma. Poisoning from acids and alkalis causes burns on the lips, mouth, and tongue. An overdose of an iron tonic produces abdominal pain and severe, often bloody vomiting, followed by collapse.

Home Treatment

Two steps are vital. First, try to determine quickly how much of the substance your child has taken and when. Second, call your doctor or a local poison control center for instructions. Read the label of the drug or other preparation over the phone. You will be advised whether or not to induce vomiting.

If your child has not vomited, if the poison was neither a strong acid nor an alkali, and if your child is conscious, induce vomiting by giving two to three teaspoonsful of syrup of ipecac followed by a half to full glass of water or juice. (**Do not give milk**.) If vomiting does not occur within 20 to 30 minutes, repeat the syrup of ipecac liquid dose. To induce vomiting may not be safe after volatile hydrocarbons have been swallowed.

Precautions

• The most important precaution is to see that all poisonous substances are stored out of reach of children—under lock and key if necessary. • Do not place or store dangerous substances in other than their original containers (for example, kerosene left in a drinking glass, medication kept in an unlabeled container). • Insist upon child-proof tops on all medicines, not just those for children. • More children are fatally poisoned by adult aspirin than by children's flavored aspirin. • Be careful with iron tablets. They taste sweet, look like candy, and can be deadly. • When visiting others' homes, do not let your children explore until you are sure there are no poisons within reach. • When guests visit you, be certain they children. • Keep the telephone numbers of the police and fire departments, your doctor, and the local poison control center near the telephone. • Always have syrup of ipecac in the house.

Doctor's Treatment

Treatment depends upon an accurate history and a thoughtful diagnosis. Only a few specific antidotes are available to reverse poisoning from among thousands of poisonous substances. Your doctor may induce vomiting with syrup of ipecac or wash out the stomach by means of a tube. Further treatment varies with the substance ingested and your child's condition.

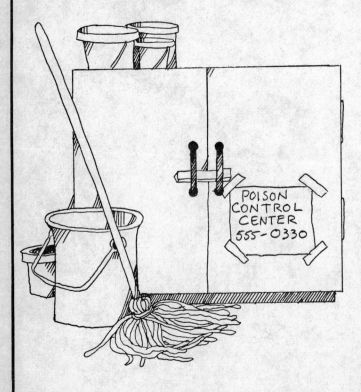

Make sure that all poisonous substances are locked away, out of reach of children.

POISON CONTROL CENTER 555-0330

Description

Also known as *poliomyelitis* and *infantile paralysis*, polio is an infection of the spinal cord that is due to three related but different viruses. Attack by each type of virus confers lifelong immunity against that type only. Therefore, it is possible to have three separate attacks of the disease.

Polio virus is found in the saliva and the stools of patients, and it is transmitted by direct contact or fecal contamination through swimming pools, toys, or food. The incubation period for polio is three to fourteen days.

Of those children who develop polio, 93 to 95 percent of them have no symptoms but develop immunity. Four to five percent of those infected develop a minor illness, with fever, malaise, sore throat, and nausea for three to four days. One to two percent develop clinically recognizable polio, with symptoms of a minor illness plus sore, stiff muscles and a stiff neck and spine. Within this one or two percent are the children who become paralyzed or die.

Diagnosis

Minor illness cases may never be recognized as polio unless they occur as part of an epidemic. Diagnosis is based on examination of viral cultures and studies of antibodies in the blood. Central nervous system involvement is suspected when an ill child has a stiff neck and back and must support himself tripod-fashion (when sitting on the floor, the child must brace himself with both arms; hence, tripod). It is confirmed by the results of a spinal tap, cultures, or antibody studies.

Home Treatment

The imperative home treatment is prevention through immunization. Oral, live virus vaccine (Sabin) is effective against all three types of polio, and it confers long-lasting immunity. The risk of paralysis from present-day vaccines is less than one in ten million—a far cry from the one in a thousand risk of exposure to naturally-occurring viruses.

Precautions

● Infants are temporarily immune to each of the three types of polio for four to six months only if their mothers are immune. A full series of oral vaccine is needed to achieve long-lasting immunity. ● Anyone who has received injections of original, dead vaccine (Salk) must have boosters or two full series of the oral vaccine to guarantee immunity. ● Polio virus still exists in this country, and polio is epidemic in many other countries of the world. Avoidance isn't possible; immunity is essential.

Doctor's Treatment

Your doctor's diagnosis will be made on the basis of a physical examination and the results of a spinal tap. A child with a suspected or known case of polio will be isolated. A child who is not immunized and has been exposed to the disease will be given gamma globulin. A child who has contracted polio will be given aspirin, acetaminophen, codeine, opiates and hot packs to reduce the pain. If he is paralyzed by the disease an artificial respirator, tracheostomies, prolonged physical therapy, braces or orthopedic surgery may be required.

Related Topics: Immunizations, Viruses

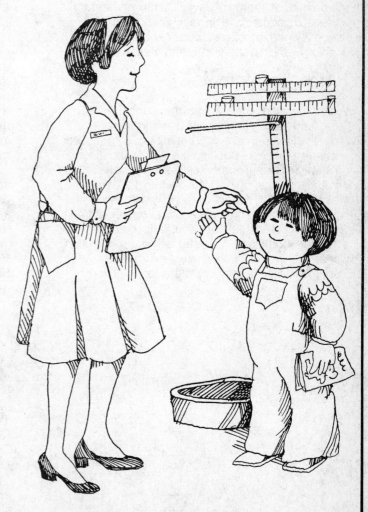

Your child needs a full series of oral polio vaccine for long-lasting immunity.

PUNCTURE WOUNDS

Description

Wounds that pierce the skin are classified as abrasions (scrapes), lacerations (cuts), and punctures. A puncture is a wound whose depth is greater than its length and width. Most puncture wounds in children are made by nails, needles, pins, knives, and splinters.

Because of their small opening and their depth, punctures have four particular dangers: the tetanus germ thrives in the absence of air, so punctures are ideal sites for developing tetanus; they are hard to clean, so punctures are susceptible to infection; punctures can penetrate deep into the body; and they may harbor foreign bodies that are difficult to detect.

Diagnosis

The presence of a puncture wound usually is obvious. The important aspects of the diagnosis involve determining whether the puncture has penetrated into a deeper structure (joint, abdominal or thoracic cavity, skull, or tendon), whether it contains a foreign body (broken needle, wood or glass splinter, or shred of clothing), and whether it is infected.

Home Treatment

Wash the skin surrounding the puncture with soap and water and apply a nonirritating (nonstinging, nonburning, noninjurious) antiseptic such as solution—not tincture—of Merthiolate antiseptic. Be sure your child's tetanus immunization is up to date (within five years). Make sure that the instrument which made the wound is intact and has not broken off at the tip. Inspect and feel the wound to determine if a foreign body can be detected under the skin. Cover the wound with a sterile bandage and inspect it twice a day for signs of infection (redness, discharge, swelling, increasing pain, and tenderness).

Precautions

• Puncture wounds in the abdomen or chest may be very serious. Be sure to take your child to a doctor. • Punctures of a joint may cause purulent arthritis within hours. The knee joint is particularly vulnerable; a puncture near a joint, especially the knee, should be seen by a doctor. Any signs of purulent arthritis (redness, swelling, increasing pain, inability to move the joint through its full range of normal motion) should be considered a **medical emergency**. • Do not remove an object even if it is a knife blade, nail, wood, glass, or needle from a puncture wound. Let your doctor remove it. Further damage can be caused by improper removal of the object. • If a puncture wound remains tender for more than one or two days, it should be seen by your doctor.

Doctor's Treatment

A puncture wound cannot be cleaned properly, even by a doctor. Your doctor will try to determine if any foreign bodies are present by feeling the wound or by X ray. Such foreign material may need to be removed surgically; or the doctor may wait and observe the wound for awhile perhaps recommending that it be soaked in Epsom salts solution for five to ten minutes four times a day. Antibiotics will be prescribed if the wound is infected, tetanus toxoid if immunization is not current. If a wound has penetrated a joint, the abdomen, chest, skull, or a tendon, your doctor will explore the wound surgically.

Related Topics: Arthritis, Cuts, Immunizations, Scrapes

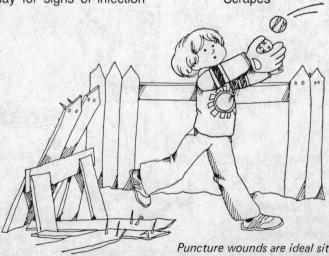

Puncture wounds are ideal sites for developing tetanus and are susceptible to infection.

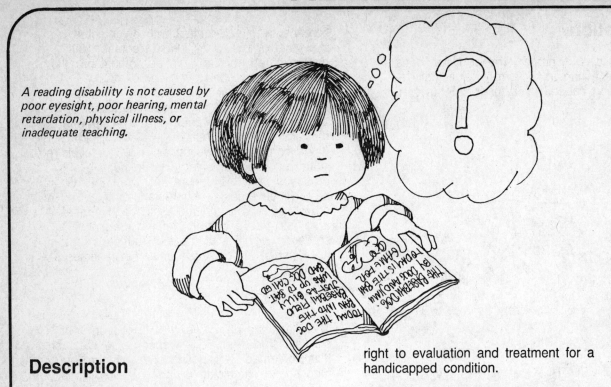

A reading disability is not caused by poor eyesight, poor hearing, mental retardation, physical illness, or inadequate teaching.

Description

Most children learn to spell and to read with understanding by the second grade. And as they age year by year, their reading ability keeps pace with their accomplishments in other school subjects. If your child has not learned to read by second grade, does not enjoy reading about things that interest him, or his reading doesn't keep pace with progress in other subjects, things should be investigated. (In older children trouble in other subjects may indicate an inability to read adequately.)

A reading disability is not caused by poor eyesight, poor hearing, physical illness, inadequate teaching, or mental retardation. Each of these conditions interferes with reading and should be detected. But none of them is a true reading disability.

Diagnosis

Five to twenty-five percent of the children in the United States have a reading disability, which may be inborn and common to several members of the family.

A reading problem should be suspected if your child at or above the second-grade level avoids reading for pleasure, even when other forms of entertainment—play or television—are unavailable, and if achievement test scores in reading are consistently below test scores in other subjects. A firm understanding of your child's reading ability can be achieved by having a battery of tests administered by a trained educational psychologist. Check with school officials concerning your child's legal right to evaluation and treatment for a handicapped condition.

Home Treatment

The important home treatment is to be aware of the problem and to refrain from assuming that a child who is not learning to read is "lazy."

Precautions

● Expect your child to enjoy reading by the second grade. ● Read to him at home to encourage a familiarity and love of books. ● Obtain your child's test scores each time the tests are administered (every two years in many school systems). ● If you suspect that your child is having trouble learning to read, consult school personnel and your doctor for advice.

Doctor's Treatment

Your doctor will conduct a complete physical examination, including vision and hearing. The doctor can also help you assess school records and test scores and refer you to a learning specialist who will evaluate your child's academic strengths and weaknesses. A learning specialist or a doctor then should plan your child's educational program with school personnel to take advantage of his abilities and make allowances for his difficulties.

Related Topics: Deafness, Hyperactivity, Vision (These chapters should be read so you are aware of what physical conditions may be affecting your child's reading.)

RINGWORM

Description

Ringworm is a misnomer. The condition does not involve a ring or a worm. It is actually a skin infection caused by a fungus. Ringworm

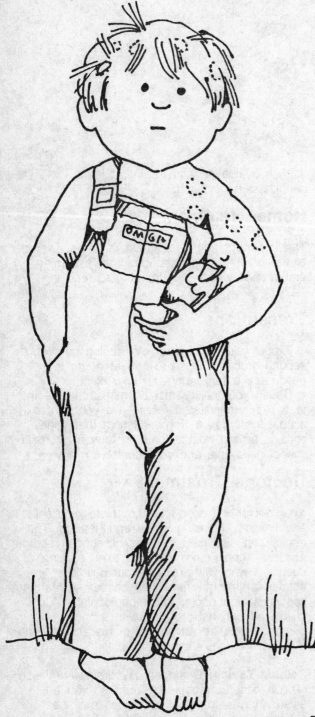

spreads by direct contact with an infected individual or pet or by indirect contact with contaminated objects such as combs, pillows, towels, clothing, and even floors.

Different funguses prefer different areas of the body. Ringworm of the scalp (tinea capitis) appears as scaly patches on the scalp with stubs of broken-off hairs. Ringworm of the body (tinea corporis) shows up as round or oval, red, scaly patches that enlarge while healing proceeds from the center. Ringworm of the groin (tinea cruris) is characterized by a red or brown, scaly rash on the crotch and genital area and has a sharply defined margin of spread. Ringworm of the feet (athlete's foot; tinea pedis) affects the feet and sometimes the ankles and legs.

Diagnosis

The diagnosis of ringworm is based on your child's history and close inspection of the rash. It is confirmed by isolating and culturing the fungus and examining it under a microscope.

Home Treatment

Fungicidal ointments such as Whitfield's, haloprogin, chlortrimazole, tolnaftate, and undecylenic acid ointments are applied until the skin clears.

Precautions

● Several other common rashes resemble ringworm. If a rash does not improve after several days of home treatment see your doctor. ● Treatment of ringworm may create its own rash on sensitive skin. If the rash worsens or changes in character stop home treatment and see your doctor.

Doctor's Treatment

Your doctor can validate your diagnosis by viewing your child's rash under ultraviolet light and by culturing and microscopically examining the results. A local fungicidal ointment or an oral fungicide such as griseofulvin fungicide may be prescribed.

Related Topic: Athlete's Foot (Also be familiar with other rashes described in this book so you may distinguish one from the other and provide proper treatment.)

Ringworm is not a worm, but an infection caused by a fungus.

ROCKY MOUNTAIN SPOTTED FEVER

Description

Rocky Mountain spotted fever is an acute, noncontagious rash and fever which is transmitted by the bite of a wood, rabbit, or dog tick. The name of the disease is misleading since it is just as common in Virginia, Delaware, and Maryland as in the Rocky Mountain states and occurs in all states.

The disease is caused by a microorganism called rickettsia that is midway between a virus and a bacterium. The incubation period for the disease is two to eight days. It starts with vague symptoms of headache, fever, and loss of appetite. One to five days later, a rash appears on the ankles and wrists and spreads rapidly to involve the entire body. The rash's pale rose-colored, flat or slightly raised spots often become reddish-purple. As the disease progresses the fever worsens, and severe muscle pain develops. Usually, the illness lasts about two to three weeks if complications do not arise. As many as 40 percent of the people with Rocky Mountain spotted fever who receive no treatment die.

Diagnosis

Rocky Mountain spotted fever can be suspected if a rash and symptoms follow a tick bite. The diagnosis cannot be confirmed, however, until the second week of the illness when the antibody levels in the blood rise up against the rickettsiae.

Home Treatment

There is no home treatment except to **watch for symptoms** of Rocky Mountain spotted fever in children who are exposed to ticks. If they appear see your doctor promptly.

Precautions

● Remove ticks from dogs cautiously with tweezers, not fingers. A crushed tick can contaminate a scratch in the skin and transmit rickettsiae. ● Use tick repellents on pets. ● Do not allow your child to handle wild rabbits. ● Observe the health of your child carefully for a week following a tick bite.

Doctor's Treatment

Your doctor may begin giving your child antibiotics even before tests have confirmed Rocky Mountain spotted fever if there is strong reason to suspect it. Tetracycline and chloramphenicol are medicines used for initial treatment. Steroids are used to treat severe cases. Hospitalization for up to ten days may be advisable.

A partially effective vaccine for use against Rocky Mountain spotted fever is available, but it is not recommended for routine use. It is only advisable for those living or traveling in heavily tick-infested areas.

Related Topic: Insect Bites

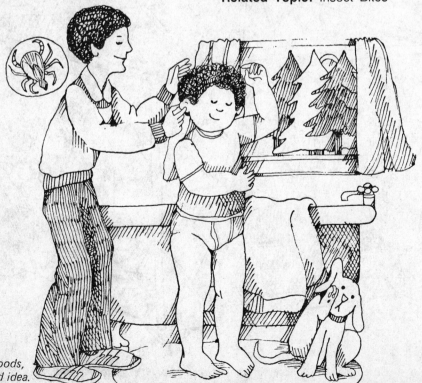

After a day in the woods, a tick check is a good idea.

ROSEOLA

Description

Roseola is an acute, infectious disease—caused by an unidentified virus—which is characterized by a high fever followed by a rash. It occurs almost exclusively in infants from six months to three years of age. The incubation period for the disease is seven to seventeen days. One attack provides lifelong immunity.

Roseola begins suddenly with a fever of 104°F to 106°F. It often causes convulsions at the onset but rarely any other symptoms. Sometimes, it causes a runny nose, mild redness of the throat, and minimal enlargement of the lymph nodes of the neck. Generally, the fever persists for three or four days and cannot be kept down with aspirin or acetaminophen. Meanwhile, your child appears to be less ill than the degree of the fever suggests. The fever disappears abruptly; at the same time, a splotchy, red rash appears on the trunk and spreads to the child's arms and neck. When the rash disappears in one or two days, your child is well again. Complications are rare.

Diagnosis

Roseola is difficult to identify until the fever drops and the rash appears. **In no other disease does a rash follow a fever.** The diagnosis is confirmed when, after one or two days, the white blood count drops below normal.

Home Treatment

Give aspirin or acetaminophen or both to help control the fever. Medication to prevent convulsions will be prescribed as needed.

Precautions

● Another common illness that produces a high fever but few other symptoms or abnormal physical findings is infection of the urinary tract. It is most common in girls. ● Coughing, vomiting, diarrhea, discharge from the eyes or ears, and prostration are NOT associated with roseola.

Doctor's Treatment

Through a careful physical examination, your doctor will rule out other illnesses which cause high fevers. A subnormal white blood cell count will be looked for after the first or second day to confirm the diagnosis.

Related Topics: Convulsions with Fever, Fever, Urinary Tract Infection

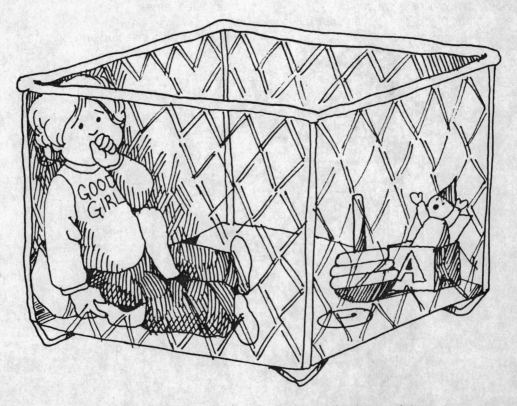

Roseola occurs almost exclusively in children under the age of three.

Description

Rubella, or German measles, is the mildest contagious disease of childhood, but it is a threat to an unborn fetus of a susceptible, pregnant woman. Women who contract rubella during the first three months of pregnancy have a 50-50 chance of delivering an infant who has cataracts, a cleft palate, an abnormal heart, or is permanently deaf or mentally deficient.

Rubella is caused by a specific virus and may be transmitted by droplets, direct contact with an infected individual, or indirect contact with articles contaminated by the secretions from the nose, throat, urine, or stools. The incubation period for the disease is 14 to 21 days. One attack confers lifelong immunity.

Characteristic symptoms of rubella are swollen, tender lymph nodes in front of and behind the ears, at the base of the skull, and on the sides of the neck. In a day or two, a fine or splotchy, dark-pink rash begins on the face; it spreads over the rest of the body within 24 hours. The rash usually lasts about three days and may or may not be accompanied by a low-grade fever (100°F, oral; 101°F, rectal), slight reddening of the throat and the whites of the eyes, and mild loss of appetite.

The patient is contagious for the period from seven days before the onset of the illness until four or five days after the appearance of the rash. Infants born with rubella may be contagious for as long as a year.

Diagnosis

No other disease causes a rash and tender enlargement of the particular lymph nodes involved in rubella. The diagnosis of rubella can be proved by isolation of the virus from the throat, blood, or urine cultures or by a rise in the blood level of antibodies against the rubella virus.

Home Treatment

Give aspirin or acetaminophen to reduce fever or discomfort. Keep your child away from pregnant women.

Precautions

● Women should be immunized against rubella, or they should receive a blood test to be certain they are immune to the disease before becoming pregnant. If they are not immune women should be immunized at least two months before trying to become pregnant. ● All children should be immunized against rubella.

● If a pregnant woman has been exposed to rubella, she should consult her obstetrician promptly.

Doctor's Treatment

Doctors do not treat rubella in children but do establish the diagnosis by means of a physical examination and certain laboratory tests. They study antibody levels to confirm the diagnosis of rubella in pregnant women.

Related Topic: Immunizations

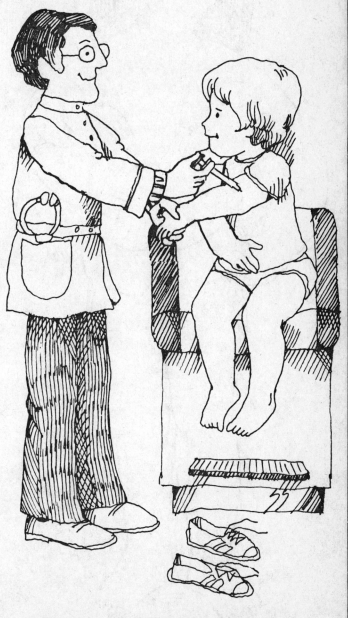

Immunization against rubella provides lifelong immunity.

SCABIES

Description

Scabies is a skin infection that is caused by the mite Sarcoptes scabei, a crawling insect barely visible to the eye. Mites burrow under the skin to lay eggs. The eggs hatch quickly, and the mites' offspring continue to tunnel until they mature in two weeks. Mature mites

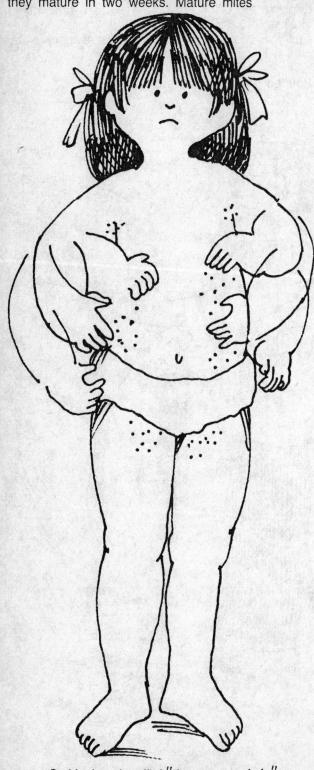

Scabies is aptly called "the seven-year itch."

congregate around hair follicles, mate, and gradually begin the cycle all over again.

Scabies is easily transmitted to others. It can be spread by direct human contact. It rarely is spread by animals.

The burrowing of the insects and the allergic reaction to their presence cause relentless itching. But scratching can result in injury to the skin or a secondary infection.

The infestation of the mites typically occurs in between the fingers and toes, on the palms of the hands and undersides of the wrists, in the armpits, at the waistline, and on the penis. Because mites may attack the skin around a woman's nipples, scabies may occur on the face of breast-fed infants.

Diagnosis

The diagnosis is based on the appearance and location of the small, red dots on the skin that mark the openings to insects' burrows. The diagnosis also is suggested by gray or black lines on the skin that mark the insects' tunnels. However, these signs on the skin can be obscured quickly by scratching.

Home Treatment

Mites can be destroyed by applying a lindane ointment or lotion (available by prescription only) or an ointment or lotion containing benzene hexachloride or crotonyl-N-ethyl-o-toluide to all skin surfaces except the head and the face. (If your infant appears to have scabies on his face consult your doctor before applying any scabicide.) All family members should receive treatment at the same time. Treatment may be repeated once or twice. Oral antihistamines may be used to alleviate itching at least temporarily.

Precautions

● If marks on the skin and itching continue after treatment, the individual may have been reinfested, or he may have a persistent allergic reaction or secondary infection. Do not keep treating the condition; see your doctor.
● Destroy mites on undergarments, bedding, and towels by laundering. ● Lindane ointment or lotion is poisonous; be sure to keep it out of the reach of children.

Doctor's Treatment

Your doctor will prescribe oral antibiotics to treat a secondary infection and antihistamines or steroids to reduce an allergic reaction.

Related Topic: Impetigo

SCHOOL PHOBIA

Description

An overwhelming fear of attending school is known as school phobia; it is not the same as truancy. A child with either problem may resort to almost anything to avoid going to and remaining in school. However, the truant child is outspoken about not wanting to attend school, is brazen about cutting classes, and is outwardly unperturbed about his absences. In contrast the child with school phobia wants to attend school, is unhappy about missing classes, and is outwardly disturbed. Without support, the school-phobic child cannot overcome his anxiety about school.

The most common cause of school phobia is separation anxiety. The child experiences uncontrollable terror when he thinks of separation from his parents and his home. Often, the child's anxiety originates from a *parent's* anxiety about separation from the child. Up to age two or three, children usually are apprehensive about separation. But as they gain experience in the world, children gradually lose this fear. Separation anxiety in a five-year-old borders on the abnormal, but it still is not uncommon and often can be easily overcome. If it continues after kindergarten, separation anxiety requires professional intervention.

Other causes of school phobia are rational fears. They include the fear of being bullied or taunted by other children, dread of a particular teacher or subject, recent death or divorce in the family, jealousy of a sibling, and guilt or fear stemming from sexual abuse within or outside the family.

Diagnosis

A child who has a mild school phobia: experiences abdominal pain and bouts of vomiting on school-day mornings; repeatedly misses the school bus; or reports to the school nurse with a headache or stomach ache soon after reaching school. In severe cases of school phobia, the child shakes, cries, and screams.

Home Treatment

The best course is to prevent the problem. By the age of two, if not earlier, your child should begin to spend brief periods of time away from both parents. No later than age three, your child should have social contact with peers without your constant supervision.

If your child in nursery school or kindergarten has school phobia remain in class with your child for a few weeks. If your presence in school does not alleviate the problem after a reasonable period of time, take your child out of school and gradually (daily) wean him from your constant presence. If your child still has school phobia after kindergarten look for the cause. If consultation with school personnel discloses grounds for rational fear (he *is* being bullied by others or he *does* dread arithmetic, for example) do all you can to alleviate these problems. If there is no apparent cause, consider the possibility that your child has a separation anxiety and seek professional help.

Precautions

● Your child must continue to attend school while the cause of the problem is sought and corrected. You may have to accompany him to and from school or allow your child to spend brief periods of time in the nurse's office or the library while there. ● Tranquilizers may be used temporarily to calm the child. They should never be used as sole treatment. Consult your doctor concerning their use.

Doctor's Treatment

Your doctor may discover the root of the problem when taking your child's health history, or it may be uncovered in consultation with school personnel, in counseling, or in psychometric testing (a technique of mental measurement). If the source of the phobia remains obscure, your doctor will recommend psychiatric counseling.

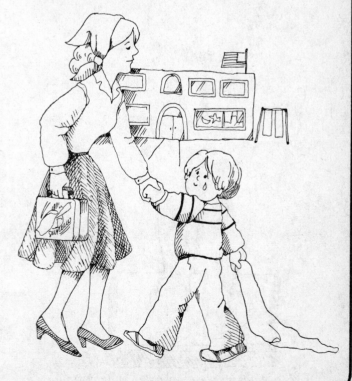

Look for emotional causes of school phobia.

SCOLIOSIS

Description

Scoliosis is also known as *curvature of the spine.* In profile a normal spine, or vertebral column, traces an S curve from top to bottom of the back; and viewed from the front or the rear, the spine is straight from side to side. In scoliosis, the vertebral column curves toward one side or the other. And that curve toward one side produces a second, compensating, curve in the spine to keep the head straight.

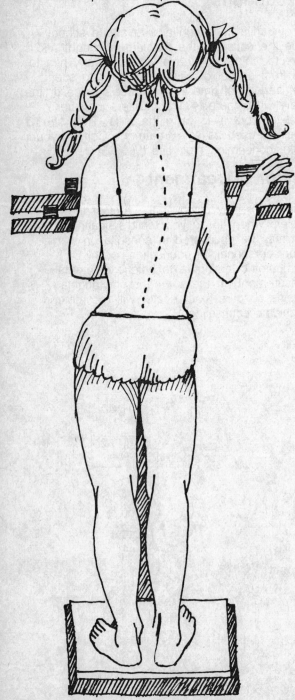

Severe scoliosis is evident when the child stands up.

One type of scoliosis (*idiopathic scoliosis*), which more frequently affects girls than boys, has no known cause. It arises during adolescence and ceases to get worse when the child stops growing. The other types of scoliosis may develop at any age, and be caused by: damage to the vertebrae due to infection; a tumor; injury; radiation therapy; abnormal development of the vertebrae or ribs; or weakness in the muscles of the trunk. Scoliosis also may result from a difference in the length of the legs. Unlike other forms of the disease, this type of scoliosis does not result in a fixed curvature of the spine; the vertebral column straightens when the child lies down.

Diagnosis

When scoliosis is severe, the curvature of the spine can easily be seen when the child stands up. Even when scoliosis is mild, the curvature may be evident because the child stands in a hip-shot position with one hip more prominent than the other. Scoliosis in almost any degree can be observed when the child bends forward with his knees straight. In this position scoliosis will cause the chest to rotate, making one side of the back more prominent.

Home Treatment

The important aspect of home treatment is to watch for the onset of the condition by observing your child's posture periodically, particularly during periods of rapid growth.

Precautions

● Any evidence of curvature of the spine is abnormal. Since scoliosis can become severe in a matter of months, your child should be checked and the condition followed by a doctor.

Doctor's Treatment

After confirming the presence of the disease, your doctor will often refer you to an orthopedist, who is skilled in treating scoliosis. The specialist will x-ray the spine. Differences in leg length will be treated by placing lifts in shoes or by surgery.

Idiopathic scoliosis occasionally corrects itself during growth. However, it must be checked several times a year. Correction of idiopathic scoliosis may require the use of a back brace or surgery of the spine.

No matter what type of scoliosis, exercise and other modes of physical therapy are not known to be helpful.

Description

A scrape (abrasion) is a shallow break in the skin caused by an injury. Scrapes are distinguished from cuts and lacerations in that their depth is less than their surface length and width. Scrapes are, certainly, the most common and least dangerous injuries sustained by children. Most of them do not involve the loss of a full thickness of skin. They therefore heal with little or no scarring. However, any embedded dirt, sand, gravel, or blacktop may be permanently sealed under the skin if it is not removed before the abrasion heals.

As long as the full thickness of the skin has not been injured, bleeding will be uneven over the entire surface of the scrape; the scrape will have large and small areas that do not bleed.

Diagnosis

Scrapes are obvious. When the surface of a scrape does not bleed uniformly, it is classified as a first- or second-degree abrasion and can be treated at home. A third-degree abrasion bleeds uniformly over its entire surface, may scar, and must be seen by a doctor.

Home Treatment

To stop the bleeding, apply gentle pressure directly to the wound through a square of sterile gauze. Wash the wound with soap and water; then, look for any embedded dirt. Inspect the wound carefully under good light and, if necessary, with a magnifying glass.

If dirt is not embedded in the wound, apply a non-stinging antiseptic, cover the scrape with a sterile bandage, and keep it covered until it heals completely and the scab falls off spontaneously. If the abrasion is in the area of constant motion (at a joint, for example), periodically swab the scab with an antibiotic or antiseptic ointment to keep it pliable and to avoid cracking.

If dirt is embedded in the wound, dab anesthetic ointment on the area for 30 to 60 minutes; then begin to scrub gently. Sometimes, residual dirt will be extruded from a wound if the abrasion is kept covered and liberal amounts of antibiotic ointment are applied twice a day.

Precautions

• Do not treat an abrasion that involves the full thickness of the skin. • Remove dirt from an abrasion, both to guard against infection and to prevent it from being permanently sealed under the skin. • Tetanus is unlikely, but not impossible. Since doctors seldom treat abrasions, keep the child's tetanus boosters up to date. • Impetigo may begin at the site of an abrasion; treat accordingly.

Doctor's Treatment

If an abrasion is deep and badly soiled your doctor will anesthetize the region and scrub out the dirt with a brush or solvent.

Related Topics: Cuts, Impetigo, Puncture Wounds

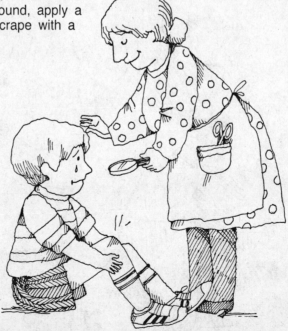

Inspect wounds carefully for embedded dirt.

SHINGLES

Description

Shingles is an acute infection that produces crops of tough blisters on the skin. Shingles is caused by the same virus that causes chicken pox; people who develop shingles have had chicken pox at some time in the past. Presumably, after a bout of chicken pox, the chicken pox-shingles virus (the varicella-zoster virus) lies dormant in the body until, for some reason, it is reactivated to cause shingles. Shingles is unusual in children under ten years of age, but it becomes increasingly more common with advancing age. One attack of shingles almost always brings lifelong immunity.

The initial symptoms of shingles are lethargy, fever, and pain and tenderness along the course of a nerve. Usually, shingles erupts on the chest, back, or abdomen, but it may occur along a nerve in the head or face, and involve an eye. In a few days red pimples appear on the skin, and nearby lymph nodes enlarge. The pimples turn into blisters which dry out and form scabs in five to ten days. New crops of pimples may continue to appear for up to a week, but the rash and pain disappear in the following one to five weeks.

Diagnosis

The diagnosis is based on the typical appearance of the rash—which is confined to the length of one or two nerves—and the pain. Before the rash appears, the pain—sometimes intense—may simulate pleurisy, or an acute abdominal condition, or heart pain. In doubtful cases diagnosis is made on the basis of the results of complicated blood tests.

Home Treatment

No treatment is helpful other than giving aspirin or acetaminophen to reduce the pain.

Precautions

● If shingles involves the eye, consult an eye specialist. ● People who have shingles may transmit chicken pox. If your child is susceptible to chicken pox and is at high risk from chicken pox (for example, if he is taking steroids, which are immunosuppressants) and is exposed to someone with shingles take him to your doctor.

Doctor's Treatment

Your doctor may prescribe steroids for shingles. He may give zoster immune globulin (ZIG) or immune serum globulin (ISG) to a child who is at risk from chicken pox and who has been exposed to shingles.

Related Topics: Chest Pain, Chicken Pox

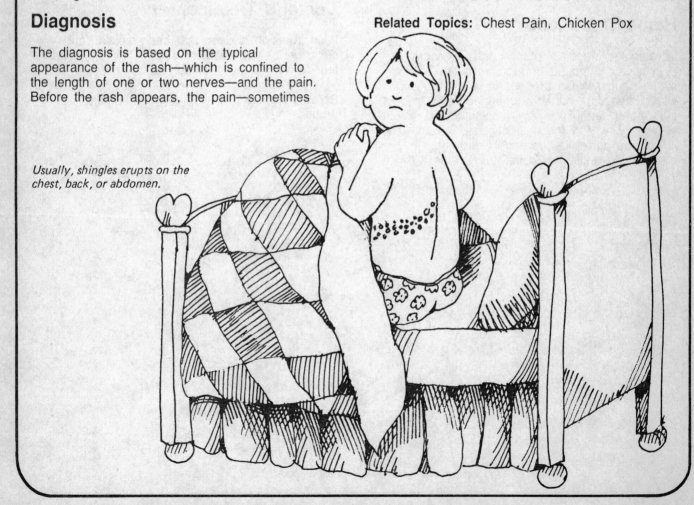

Usually, shingles erupts on the chest, back, or abdomen.

SHORTNESS OF BREATH

Description

When a child breathes, he takes in oxygen to fuel the body for action and rids the body of carbon dioxide, the end product of metabolism. When the body's demand for oxygen is not met or it retains too much carbon dioxide, shortness of breath results. Shortness of breath usually follows prolonged physical exertion, but it also may accompany fever because the elevated temperature speeds up the body's chemical reactions, which, in turn, increase the amount of carbon dioxide in the body and the demand for oxygen.

Shortness of breath also may be a sign of disease. It indicates that something is interfering with the intake and transport of oxygen. It may be due to croup; inflammation of the bronchial tubes or the epiglottis in the throat; asthma; pneumonia; inhalation of a foreign body; or spontaneous collapse of a lung (pneumothorax).

Inadequate transport of oxygen causing shortness of breath may signal the presence of heart disease, severe anemia, or carbon monoxide poisoning from automobile exhaust fumes or a defective heater.

A rapid rate of respiration may be a consequence of aspirin poisoning, which stimulates the breathing centers in the brain, or uncontrolled diabetes and dehydration. Anxiety gives the false sensation of shortness of breath.

Diagnosis

The diagnosis of shortness of breath depends on the rate of respiration. To determine if your child is actually short of breath count the number of respirations per minute when he is at rest. The average, normal rate of breathing for newborns is 40 respirations per minute; for one-year-olds, it is 30; and for those over eight years old it is 20. If the rate of respiration for your child at rest is double the normal rate, he has shortness of breath.

Your child's fever may hinder your ability to judge whether his respiration is normal. If your child seems to be short of breath and has a fever, allow two or three extra breaths per minute for each temperature degree above normal, or time his breathing after his temperature has returned to normal.

Home Treatment

Except for air hunger (anxiety), no home treatment for shortness of breath should be attempted. Ask your doctor's advice.

Precautions

● A fever increases a person's rate of breathing. If the fever is treated with aspirin and the dosage given is too high, the rate of breathing will increase even more. If your child who is taking aspirin becomes short of breath, double-check the dose of the aspirin to see if it's too high. ● Rapid respiration while your child is resting often signals a serious problem. Contact your doctor promptly whenever it occurs.

Doctor's Treatment

Your doctor will perform a complete examination paying particular attention to the lungs, heart, throat, epiglottis and blood pressure, and ordering chest and neck X rays. Blood and urine tests will be ordered to determine if the underlying cause of the shortness of breath is diabetes. Questions put to you might include whether your child has been exposed to poisonous gases or whether he is being treated with aspirin for some other health condition. The specific treatment of shortness of breath depends on its cause; it may involve hospitalization and the administration of oxygen.

Related Topics: Asthma, Breathing Difficulty, Croup, Pneumonia

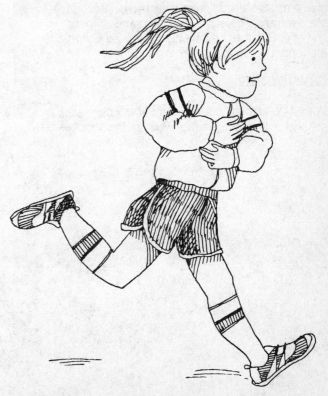

Shortness of breath following exertion is normal.

SINUSITIS

Description

Sinusitis is an inflammation or infection of the sinuses, the air-filled cavities in the face that connect with the nasal passages. Around the nose are three pairs of sinuses (the *maxillary*, *frontal*, and *ethmoid* sinuses) and one midline sinus (the *sphenoid*). The maxillary sinuses, which lie below the eyes, and the ethmoid sinuses, which are between the eyes, are present in infancy. The sphenoid sinus, located behind the roof of the nose, is fully developed between the ages of three and five years, and the frontal sinuses, situated above the eyes, at six to ten years.

Because the sinuses are continuations of the nasal cavity, they are affected by any viral infection of the nose or any allergic reaction in the nose. Sometimes, a virus or an allergy attacks the openings to the sinuses, which induces a bacterial infection within the sinus. Sometimes, a bacterial infection of the sinus follows a bacterial infection of the nose. And a bacterial infection of the sinus is true sinusitis.

The symptoms of sinusitis include fever (sometimes as high as 105°F), pain, stuffy nose, and cough. Depending on the location of the infection, headache may occur in the back of the head (infection of the sphenoid sinus), at the temples and over the eyes (infection of the ethmoid and frontal sinuses), or above and below the eyes (infection of the maxillary sinuses). Small children who have infection in the ethmoid sinus develop red and swollen eyelids. But the key to identifying sinusitis is the opaque discharge from the nose.

Diagnosis

With sinusitis, discharge from the nose is yellow, milky, or opaque. Pus in the sinuses can be revealed through X ray, but a thickening of the lining of the sinuses from a common cold or an allergy may be confused with it.

Home Treatment

The sinuses may be protected from infection by treating a cold with oral decongestants and nose drops or by treating an allergy with oral antihistamines. Decongestants, nose drops, and antihistamines also encourage drainage after sinusitis has developed. Heat may be applied to the affected sinuses, and aspirin or acetaminophen may be given to relieve the pain and fever.

Precautions

● A high fever (103°F, orally or 104°F, rectally) plus signs of sinusitis indicate a potentially serious infection. See your doctor. ● Pus-like discharge or signs of sinusitis on one side of the nose suggest a foreign object may be lodged in the nose or the nose may be deformed. See your doctor.

Doctor's Treatment

Your doctor may prescribe oral antibiotics after identifying the infecting bacteria. Suction may be used to drain the sinuses of older children with sinusitis. Surgical drainage is rarely indicated in children.

Related Topics: Allergy, Common Cold, Headaches

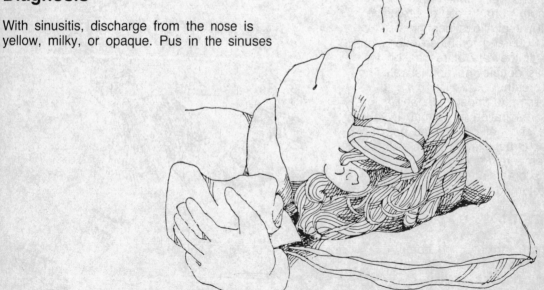

Home treatment of sinusitis can include the application of heat to the affected sinuses.

Description

Painful heels are a common complaint before and during adolescence. Almost 90 percent of the time the pain is due to injury of the bony growth plate near the back of the heel bone (calcaneus). The injury is called *Sever's disease* and may be due to a direct blow caused by heels pounding the ground or to a pull of the calf muscles on the Achilles tendon and the back of the heel bone. One or both heels hurt when walking and are tender to the touch on both sides and the bottom of the heel bone (about one-half to one inch away from the back of the heel). The heels are not swollen or red; the skin over the heels shows no abnormality.

Other problems that cause pain at the heel also cause other symptoms. For example, *osteomyelitis* (infection of the heel bone) produces severe pain that intensifies over time, red and swollen heels, and a low-grade (100°F, orally or 101°F, rectally) fever. Blisters, plantar warts, and wounds of the heel can also cause sore heels.

Diagnosis

The diagnosis of Sever's disease will be based on the presence of pain and tenderness at the heel and the absence of other symptoms.

Home Treatment

To relieve the pain from Sever's disease pad the heels of all of your child's shoes with a quarter-inch heel pad, and temporarily restrict activities that involve running and jumping. Even if an adolescent has pain in only one heel be sure to pad the heels of both shoes.

Precautions

● If your teenager can't move the affected foot up and down (by rising on tiptoes) he may have a torn Achilles tendon. **Do not attempt home care.** ● With the proper home treatment Sever's disease should subside in four to six weeks, but pain should cease as soon as the heels of the shoes are padded. If relief doesn't occur promptly take your teenager to your doctor. ● Pain may recur following a new injury. Don't worry, just repeat the treatment.

Doctor's Treatment

After a careful examination to rule out other causes of pain, your doctor will follow the same steps as you do in home treatment. Your doctor will immobilize the ankles if the case of Sever's disease is severe. X ray is seldom required.

Related Topic: Warts

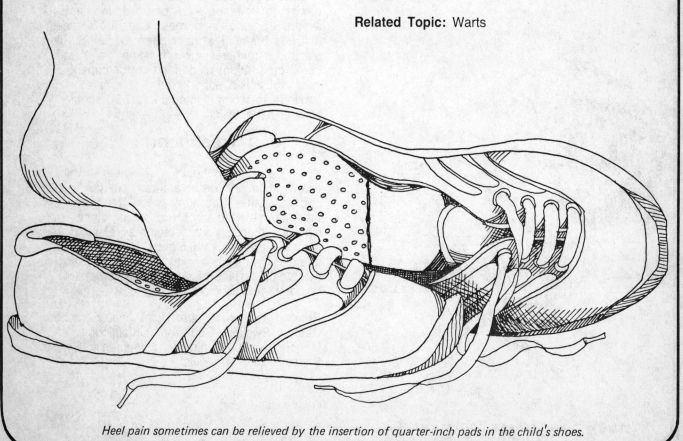

Heel pain sometimes can be relieved by the insertion of quarter-inch pads in the child's shoes.

SORE THROAT

Description

In *theory* and in the medical school classroom a sore throat is the simplest problem to diagnose and to treat. Medical textbooks state that a sore throat is usually caused by a virus and, therefore, does not require treatment with antibiotics. A sore throat that is not caused by a virus is due to streptococcus. Streptococcus organisms can be isolated on a throat culture, and a strep throat can be treated with penicillin or with erythromycin if the child is allergic to penicillin.

In *practice* the diagnosis and treatment of a sore throat is not so straightforward. Viral infections sometimes are complicated by streptococcal infections. A throat culture may isolate streptococci organisms even though the illness is not being caused by these organisms, and five to ten percent of the throat cultures will not show streptococci even when they are the cause of the sore throat. Some bacterial illnesses that cause a sore throat will respond to antibiotics, but the infecting bacteria cannot be identified on an ordinary throat culture plate.

Diagnosis

Determining the presence of a sore throat in infants and toddlers is difficult because they cannot communicate, but swollen glands in the neck or difficulty swallowing are clues. Determining the cause of a sore throat depends on the results of a throat or other type of culture, on a complete blood count, and on the doctor's skill in performing the physical examination, knowledge of the illnesses that are prevalent in the community, and professional judgment.

Home Treatment

Older children may gargle with warm salt water, but all children should drink extra fluids and eat their usual diet if they can. Give aspirin or acetaminophen to reduce pain or fever and isolate the child from other children, particularly infants, until the cause of the problem is found.

Precautions

● Take the child to a doctor if a sore throat is accompanied by any of the following symptoms: moderately or severely swollen and tender neck glands; difficulty swallowing that cannot be relieved by aspirin or acetaminophen; pus-like discharge from the eyes or nose; moderate or severe earache; tenderness over the sinuses; difficulty breathing; chest pain; reddish-purple rash or a rash resembling scarlet fever; stiff neck; prostration; disorientation; or continual vomiting. ● If a sore throat and a fever continue to worsen after 24 to 36 hours, consult a doctor.

Doctor's Treatment

Your doctor will conduct a complete physical examination and order a throat culture and, perhaps, other laboratory tests. Depending on the results of the throat culture or other laboratory tests, your doctor may elect to treat a sore throat with antibiotics. Regardless of the treatment prescribed, you should report any new symptoms or lack of improvement after 24 hours to your doctor.

Related Topics: Croup; Diphtheria; Earaches; Glands, Swollen; Gonorrhea; Infectious Mononucleosis; Meningitis; Pneumonia; Sinusitis; Strep Throat; Tonsillitis

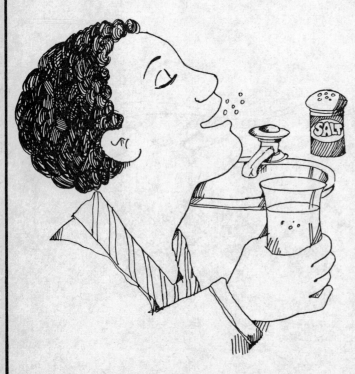

Gargling with warm salt water provides some relief.

SPEECH PROBLEMS & STUTTERING

Description

Children learn to speak by imitation. But they may learn at different rates depending on their intelligence, hearing, and their control of the muscles involved in speaking. And speech may be delayed or impaired if their speech centers in the brain or their larynx, throat, nose, tongue, or lips are not normal.

Learning to speak depends on how often a child hears speech, how well he is motivated to speak, and how much he is encouraged to speak. On the average a baby begins to babble and make letter-like sounds at four to six months of age. By eight months, he has achieved a typical baby vocabulary using such "words" as "goo," "ba-ba," and "da-da." By 12 months, a baby will be using two-syllable "words" meaningfully ("ma-ma" for mother, "ba-ba" for bottle), and by two years old will be connecting words purposefully ("go bye-bye," "want cookie.") A child of five years can speak five-word sentences, and a child of six can make all the sounds of the alphabet, except perhaps the sounds for s and z.

Children from age two to five often lack fluency, and they may stutter or stammer at times. If the lack of fluency or stuttering or stammering continues the child may have a speech problem. Or if the speech does not develop normally it may be due to partial or complete deafness, mental retardation, inadequate exposure to language, brain damage, anatomical abnormalities, or malfunction of the speech centers (aphasia).

Diagnosis

Any marked delay in a child's achieving speech raises the suspicion of a speech problem.

Home Treatment

To learn to speak adequately, your baby must be spoken to *and* listened to. Improper speech should be corrected, but a child should not be chastised, deliberately ignored, or forced to practice speaking. Stuttering in children aged two to five may be disregarded unless it is still a problem several months after its onset. It should not provoke anger or anxiety, suggestions that the child speak more slowly or more clearly, or laughter and taunts from siblings. Stuttering warrants professional attention if it is severe, constant, or prolonged.

Precautions

● If your child's speech does not develop more or less in accordance with the timetable above consult your doctor. ● Do not refuse to understand your child or to force him to speak more clearly. ● Do not call the child's attention to his stuttering. Read, sing, and speak to your child whenever possible. Notice if your child speaks only in a monotone or with a marked nasal quality or if his vocabulary and his ability to pronounce words is diminishing instead of improving.

Doctor's Treatment

Your doctor will perform a complete physical examination, checking the throat, palate, and tongue and testing your child's hearing. If your child is under the age of five you may be referred to a speech pathologist for evaluation and treatment if: stuttering is severe, constant, or unduly prolonged; the child seems to be severely frustrated; or if you need assistance in handling your child's development of speech. If your child substitutes sounds or stutters after the age of five or six, your doctor may suggest he be seen by a speech specialist.

Related Topic: Deafness

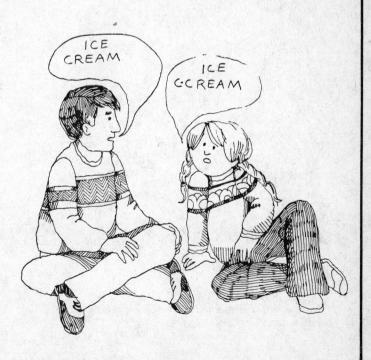

Children who stutter after the age of five may need to see a speech specialist.

SPRAINS & DISLOCATIONS

Description

All joints of the body are surrounded by ligaments, which can be partially or completely torn when the joint is forcibly twisted beyond its normal range of motion. A partially or completely torn ligament is called a *sprain*, and it causes pain (sometimes severe), swelling, tenderness, decreased motion of the joint, and internal bleeding.

If ligaments are badly torn the bones of the joint may slip out of position or become dislocated. Besides the usual symptoms of a sprain, a *dislocation* causes gross deformity and marked or total loss of function of the dislocated parts. Even after the dislocation has been corrected the joint remains unstable for weeks.

Sprains are common during childhood, but dislocations other than a dislocated elbow (Malgaigne's subluxation of the elbow) are rare.

Sprains most often occur in the fingers (called "jammed" or "baseball" fingers), toes, ankles, neck, and back. Dislocations can also occur in the fingers, toes, kneecaps, and shoulders.

Diagnosis

Because dislocations produce gross deformity, they seldom are missed. Sprains, if mild or moderate, generally can be suspected if a joint is tender after it has been twisted or overextended. Fractures of the bones of the involved joint cannot be ruled out without X rays.

Home Treatment

A dislocation should not be treated at home. Mild sprains, particularly of the fingers, toes, and ankles, may be treated safely at home by splinting and avoiding use of the involved hand or foot. The sprained part should be elevated, and cold compresses can be applied for one to four hours after injury to minimize swelling. Aspirin or acetaminophen will temporarily relieve pain. If a sprain does not improve rapidly a bone may be fractured; the child should be seen by a doctor.

Precautions

● Do not attempt to correct a dislocation, even of the fingers. Dislocations are often accompanied by a fracture. ● An apparently sprained wrist in a child actually may be a fracture of the forearm bones near the joint and a sprained thumb actually may be a fractured navicular bone. ● A severe sprain may take as long as a fracture to heal and if it is not treated properly can result in a permanently weak joint. ● A sprain is not healed if it is still swollen or if it is painful to move. ● Elastic bandages do not adequately support or protect a sprained ankle.

Doctor's Treatment

Your doctor will carefully examine all the anatomical parts of the injured joint and take X rays if a dislocation or a bad sprain is suspected. A minor sprain may be x-rayed or the joint immobilized and its rate of healing observed. If the rate of healing is not rapid enough an X ray will be ordered.

Related Topics: Dislocated Elbow, Dislocated Hips, Fractures

Treatment for a sprained joint may include elevation and immobilization.

STOMACH ACHE, ACUTE

Description

The abdomen contains the stomach, small and large intestines, liver, spleen, pancreas, kidneys, urinary bladder, gall bladder, and the organs of reproduction. Disease or injury of any of these organs can cause abdominal pain. Consequently, a "stomach ache" can test the diagnostic mettle of a parent or a doctor.

Fortunately, almost all stomach aches in children are caused by one of four problems: constipation, acute gastrointestinal upset (caused by viruses, bacteria, or dietary indiscretion), emotional stress, or urinary tract infection.

Other less frequent causes of a stomach ache are: appendicitis, acute abdominal pain from pneumonia, mononucleosis, and hepatitis.

Diagnosis

The diagnosis first involves ruling out appendicitis. If appendicitis can be ruled out, then consider that:

Your child probably is *constipated* if he has not had a bowel movement or has had a hard one recently; if the pain is intermittent (crampy) on the left side of the body and follows eating; and if the abdomen is soft and not tender.

Your child probably has *gastrointestinal upset* if he has been exposed to someone else who has acute gastroenteritis or if he has eaten too much; if the pain is intermittent and occurs around the upper abdomen, or umbilicus; or if diarrhea follows vomiting.

Your child's stomach ache is probably due to *emotional stress* if he is or has been upset and if the pain does not worsen.

If your child's pain cannot be explained by any of these causes take him to your doctor.

Your child's stomach ache probably is due to *urinary tract infection* if the pain is low in the belly or generalized and intermittent; or if he has a fever and frequent, painful urination.

Home Treatment

Treat constipation with an enema or a suppository. Unless severe (acute pain lasting for more than 24 hours), gastrointestinal upset will go away on its own, but an antiemetic can relieve the vomiting, and mild heat applied to the abdomen can relieve the pain. A stomach ache due to emotional stress will ease with relief from the stress, but one that arises from urinary tract infection requires the attention of a physician. If stomach pain persists or worsens take your child to your doctor.

Precautions

● Never give a child a laxative or place ice on the abdomen to treat abdominal pain. ● Steady, worsening pain usually is more serious than intermittent, crampy pain; but severe, regular, crampy pain may indicate a serious problem, particularly if it accompanies blood or mucus in the stools. ● Abdominal pain that forces a child to bend forward as he walks is a cause for concern. ● Abdominal pain combined with a fever and a cough suggests pneumonia. ● Severe, worsening abdominal pain that follows an injury to the abdomen or lower chest suggests internal injury.

Doctor's Treatment

Your doctor's first task is to determine the cause of the pain by taking a detailed history, performing a complete physical examination, and (often) conducting a battery of laboratory tests or X rays. If the diagnosis remains doubtful your doctor may observe your child for a few hours or ask for a consultation with another physician.

Related Topics: Appendicitis; Constipation; Dysentery; Food Poisoning; Hepatitis; Infectious Mononucleosis; Intestinal Flu; Pneumonia; Shingles; Strep Throat; Stomach Ache, Chronic; Vomiting

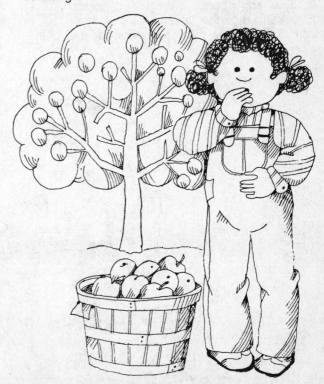

Too many green apples can cause acute stomach pain.

STOMACH ACHE, CHRONIC

Description

Intermittent abdominal pain is quite common and may continue for weeks, months, or years. In some cases the pain occurs as often as two or three times a day; in others as infrequently as two or three times a year. Of course, an attack of recurrent stomach ache may seem to be a bout of acute abdominal pain, and some conditions that cause abdominal pain may occur over and over again. However, chronic stomach pain usually is due to constipation, intolerance of cow's milk (lactase deficiency), or emotional stress. Other, less common causes are: urinary tract problems (obstruction, chronic infection); peptic ulcer; sickle cell anemia; lead poisoning; ulcerative colitis; regional enteritis (Crohn's disease); tumors; ovarian problems; worm infestations (pinworms, Giardia); intolerance of foods other than milk; and internal hernias.

Diagnosis

Recurrent abdominal pain is not due to appendicitis. To pinpoint its cause recurrent abdominal pain must be associated with other symptoms such as: vomiting; diarrhea; constipation; blood or mucus in the stools; fever; failure to gain weight; painful urination; ingesting inedible substances (pica); or anemia. Also important is the pattern of the pain—where it is, how long it lasts, and when it occurs.

In general recurrent abdominal pain that is accompanied by no other symptoms or that has no set pattern is probably not serious.

Home Treatment

If constipation is the cause of the pain correct it by giving your child an enema or a suppository. If lactase deficiency is the cause eliminate milk and milk products (cheese, yogurt, ice cream, custard) from the diet for one or two weeks; then add milk to the diet again and observe the effects. If emotional stress is responsible try to eliminate the stress. Most important, note and record the pattern of recurrent abdominal pain and any other symptoms which occur before consulting your doctor.

Precautions

● Recurrent abdominal pain from emotional stress is real and requires treatment just as much as the pain of an ulcer, ileitis, or colitis.

Doctor's Treatment

Your doctor will take a careful history of your child's recent health and perform a complete physical examination. A urinalysis and urine culture, blood tests, and stool examinations will often be ordered. If the cause of the pain still is not clear, X rays of the stomach, large and small bowels, and the urinary tract may be required. If X rays provide no clues to the problem your child may be hospitalized for extensive blood tests and internal abdominal examination (endoscopy or laparostomy).

Related Topics: Anemia; Constipation; Hernia; Pinworms; Stomach Ache, Acute; Ulcers; Urinary Tract Infections

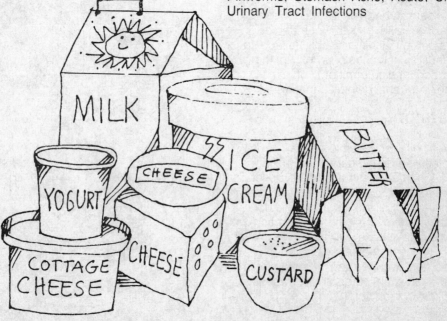

A frequent cause of chronic stomach aches is an intolerance of milk and milk products.

Description

Strep throat is a highly contagious infection of the throat usually due to the group A strain of beta-hemolytic streptococci. Although some strep germs do not cause rashes, most types can produce a toxin that causes the rash that typifies *scarlet fever* (also commonly called *scarlatina*). There are at least 60 different types of streptococcus organisms. After an attack of strep throat the individual is immune to further attack from that one type of streptococcus organism only. But once a person has had strep with a rash, he is immune to the rash for a lifetime. With or without a rash, strep throat is a serious illness.

The incubation period of strep throat is two to five days, and it is passed from child to child through the oral or nasal secretions from an infected individual, or it may be spread by a carrier who has no symptoms of the illness. At times, as many as half the children in any one area may be carriers of the disease.

The onset of strep throat is sudden. It begins with a headache, fever up to 104°F, sore and spotted throat, vomiting, abdominal pain, swollen lymph nodes in the neck, and prostration. If the infecting organism is rash-producing and the child is not immune, he will develop a rash within 24 or 72 hours. The rash is typical with fine, slightly raised, red spots resembling coarse red sandpaper. It appears on the base on the neck, in the armpits and groin, and then on the trunk and extremities. The child's face is flushed, but his lips are pale. When the rash subsides in three to twenty days, the skin flakes and peels.

A streptococcal infection **can be serious.** Among its complications are rheumatic fever, nephritis, middle ear infection, sinusitis, pneumonia, and transient arthritis.

Diagnosis

The diagnosis of a strep throat cannot be confirmed without a throat culture that isolates streptococcus organisms. However, cultures are only 90 to 95 percent reliable. The diagnosis of scarlet fever is based on the appearance of the rash.

Home Treatment

No home treatment is recommended except to alleviate the pain and fever by means of aspirin or acetaminophen. Streptococcal infections should be treated by your doctor.

Precautions

● Infants are immune to the scarlet fever toxin for four to six months if their mothers are immune. They are NOT immune to a streptococcal infection, which may be very serious but may not produce typical symptoms. Consequently, keep infants away from groups of children, some of whom may be carriers of streptococci. ● If one child in your family has a streptococcal infection watch your other children for signs of infection. ● Follow the full course of antibiotic therapy prescribed by a doctor, giving your child the medication until it is gone.

Doctor's Treatment

Strep throat is diagnosed by means of a physical examination and the results of a culture. Penicillin (or another antibiotic for those who are allergic to penicillin) is usually prescribed for ten days to cure the streptococcal infection. Antibiotics prevent rheumatic fever and *may* prevent nephritis. A child who develops complications may have to be hospitalized.

Related Topics: Arthritis, Nephritis, Pneumonia, Sinusitis, Sore Throat

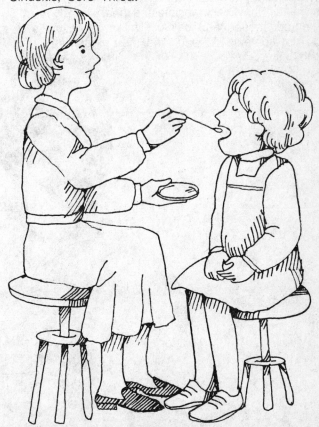

To help diagnose a strep throat a doctor will take a throat culture to determine the presence of streptococci.

STYES

Description

Styes are boils of the oil or sweat glands in the upper or lower eyelids. Usually, they are caused by staphylococcus organisms, and they may spread from individual to individual through direct contact. Styes tend to occur in crops because their pus contains staphylococci that may infect other glands in the eyelids.

Styes develop like boils. The area at the edge of the eyelid becomes increasingly red, painful, tender, and swollen. After two to three days, pus forms, and the stye "points"; that is, a yellow head appears at the edge of the lid near the base of the eyelashes. Styes usually break spontaneously, drain, and heal. Occasionally, a stye will heal without pointing or draining.

Diagnosis

Styes differ from insect bites and cysts because they are painful, tender swellings near the margins of the eyelids that usually come to a head. Insect bites itch, are not painful and do not come to a head. Cysts are lumps or swellings that show through the under surface of the eyelids as pink or pale-yellow spots. They usually are not tender. Sometimes, however, they become infected and, like styes, are red, tender, and painful. Unlike styes, cysts do not come to a head, and they persist for some time.

Home Treatment

Place warm soaks (using cotton balls or a wash cloth) on the eyelids several times a day for ten to twenty minutes each time. Give aspirin or acetaminophen to reduce pain. Administer antibiotic eye drops several times a day to prevent the formation of additional sytes. Do not treat cysts unless they are infected; then, treat them in the same way you would a stye.

Precautions

● The whites of the eyes do not become red as a result of a stye. ● One large or several small, recurring styes, or a stye that accompanies such symptoms as fever, headache, loss of appetite, or lethargy, should be seen by a doctor. ● Styes are somewhat contagious. Keep infected child's towel and washcloth separate.

Doctor's Treatment

To treat one large or several small, recurring styes, your doctor may prescribe antibiotics. A style will rarely be incised and drained. A culture of the nose and throat may be taken to ascertain the source of the staphylococci. As a last resort, your doctor may administer an immunization against staphylococci each week.

Your doctor may surgically remove an infected cyst. However, cysts often disappear spontaneously in months or years. Your doctor will treat an infected cyst the same way a stye is treated.

Related Topics: Boils, Conjunctivitis

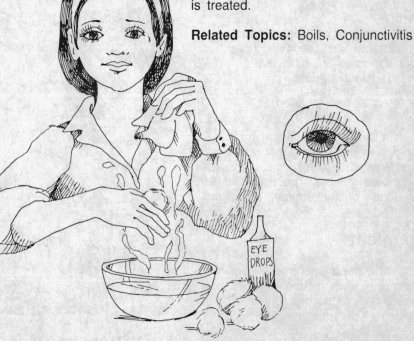

Treat styes with warm soaks on the eyelids.

Description

Sunburn is a thermal burn, usually of the first-degree. Occasionally, a sunburn causes a skin rash which resembles hives or poison ivy. This condition is called sun poisoning. Babies and children who have fair complexions are particularly susceptible to sunburn, even on cloudy days or in shade.

Diagnosis

The diagnosis of sunburn generally is immediately obvious. Sun poisoning, however, may not appear for several days.

Home Treatment

Apply cocoa butter, commercial burn ointments, cold water compresses, or a baking-soda-and-tap-water paste to the burn. Do not break blisters. Give aspirin or acetaminophen to relieve pain and antihistamines to reduce itching.

Precautions

• The most important aspect of home treatment is prevention. To tan, a child should begin slowly and gradually increase his length of exposure to the sun. • Apply sunscreens to filter out damaging rays of the sun, but remember that sunscreens do not permit unlimited exposure.

Select a sunscreen for children that includes para-aminobenzoic acid (PABA), titanium dioxide, methyl anthranilate, or sulisobenzone. And remember that all sunscreens wash off with swimming and perspiration. Follow the instructions on the product's package for reapplying the sunscreen. • Sunscreens may cause a mild rash on some people. If a rash appears, switch to another product. • Infants and children may receive a severe burn from the sun coming through the windows. Be sure children are protected by sunscreens.
• Medication applied to large sunburn areas (anesthetics in burn ointments or steroids) may be absorbed into the body and produce side effects. Use such medication sparingly. • Injury to the skin from overexposure to ultraviolet light from sunlamps is common among teenagers.
• Some medications (for example, tetracycline and its derivatives, chlorpromazine, griseofulvin and coal tar ointments) increase the sensitivity of the skin to sunburn. • Take the child to a doctor if he has a sunburn plus a fever or prostration.

Doctor's Treatment

Your doctor may prescribe oral or spray steroids to treat your child's sunburn or sun poisoning. A child who has a severe burn will be hospitalized for treatment.

Related Topic: Burns

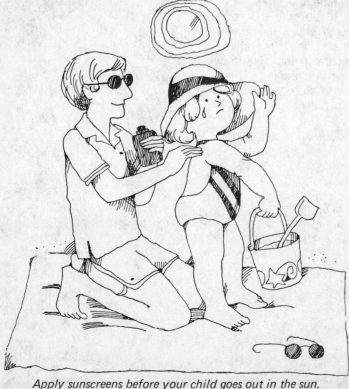

Apply sunscreens before your child goes out in the sun.

SWALLOWED OBJECTS

Description

Over 95 percent of the penny-, nickel-, or dime-size foreign objects that are swallowed by children cause no trouble and pass from the body in the stools. But objects that are the size of a quarter or larger may become lodged in the esophagus; sharp objects (pins, needles, bones, match-sticks, nails, glass splinters) may lodge in the tonsils, throat, or esophagus; and objects longer than a toothpick may not be able to pass out of the stomach.

Depending on where the object is lodged, it may cause gagging, pain, or discomfort in the throat or chest, or difficulty swallowing. Once a foreign object passes into the stomach, it does not produce any symptoms unless it obstructs or penetrates the digestive tract. Then, abdominal pain, vomiting, and fever may develop.

Diagnosis

Metallic objects are visible on an X ray, but those made of wood, plastic, or glass are not. Usually, however, the diagnosis is suggested by the circumstances and whatever symptoms of the above there may be.

Home Treatment

No treatment is necessary if the swallowed object is small and smooth. If the object is long, sharp, or large, examine the stools carefully for several days to be sure it has passed from the body. Each bowel movement must be passed through a seive. If the child has been potty trained, place in the toilet bowl a basin fashioned of window screening. Then, after the child has passed a stool wash it through the screening with hot water.

Precautions

● An object lodged in the esophagus must be removed within hours preferably by a doctor. ● No known food, drink, or medication will accelerate or make safer the passage of a foreign object through the body. ● If an object has not passed from the child's body within one week, notify your doctor. ● Try to bring a duplicate of the object when consulting your doctor. ● Do not give your child a laxative until the object has passed.

Doctor's Treatment

Your doctor will carefully inspect the throat and observe the way your child swallows. X rays of the throat, neck, chest, or abdomen may be ordered. If an object is wedged in the throat or esophagus, your doctor will remove it with an instrument. If it is in the stomach he will monitor the child's condition for three or more weeks before trying to remove it surgically. If the object is in the intestines and does not pass in one week the doctor may remove it surgically.

Related Topic: Choking

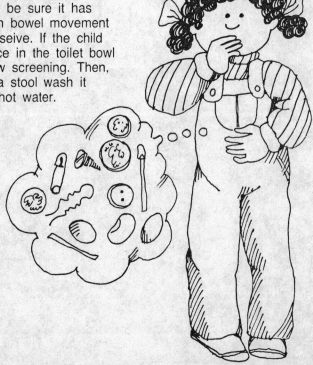

If the swallowed object is small and blunt, it will usually cause no problem.

SWIMMER'S EAR

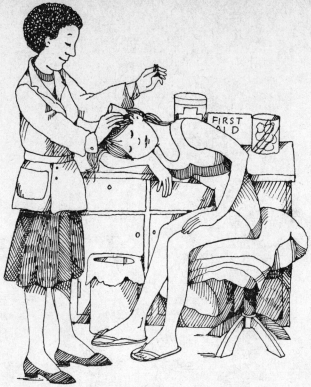

Your doctor will treat a mild case of swimmer's ear with ear drops containing antibiotics or steroids.

Description

Irritation or infection of the external ear canal is known as swimmer's ear. Swimmer's ear may arise from a middle ear infection which has caused the eardrum to rupture and pus to drain into the external canal. Or it may follow an injury to the ear canal which has become infected. Usually, however, it develops from swimming in fresh water or pools. Frequent and sustained moisture in the ear softens, swells, and cracks the ear canal and allows germs to penetrate and bring on infection.

A mild case of swimmer's ear may appear as an itching, clogged ear canal with or without odorous discharge; hearing may be diminished. A severe case may induce intense pain, fever, and swollen and tender lymph nodes in front of, behind, and below the ear.

Diagnosis

The presence of discharge in or oozing out of the ear canal suggests swimmer's ear. Without discharge from the ear, the diagnosis is based on internal examination of the ear.

Home Treatment

With your doctor's direction, administer ear drops containing antibiotics and steroids four times a day to treat a mild case of swimmer's ear. Give aspirin or acetaminophen or apply heat to the outside of the ear to reduce pain. If your child has had several bouts of swimmer's ear, drying the ear canals at the end of each day of swimming by instilling a few drops of rubbing alcohol or glycerine may prevent swimmer's ear.

Precautions

● If a child has severe pain, fever, or swollen glands, or if he does not respond to home treatment in a few days, take him to your doctor. ● Rubber earplugs will not keep water out of the ear canals. But earplugs fashioned at home from lamb's wool and coated with petroleum jelly may. ● Do not clean ear canals by using bobby pins, swabs, or anything other than a fingertip covered with a facecloth. ● If ear drops do not penetrate deeply into the ear canal, they will not be effective. After administering the drops, be sure to keep the child's head tilted.

Doctor's Treatment

In addition to ear drops your doctor may prescribe oral antibiotics. The ear canal will be cleaned if the ear is not too tender. A child who has a severe case of swimmer's ear will be hospitalized.

Related Topics: Draining Ear, Earaches

TEETHING

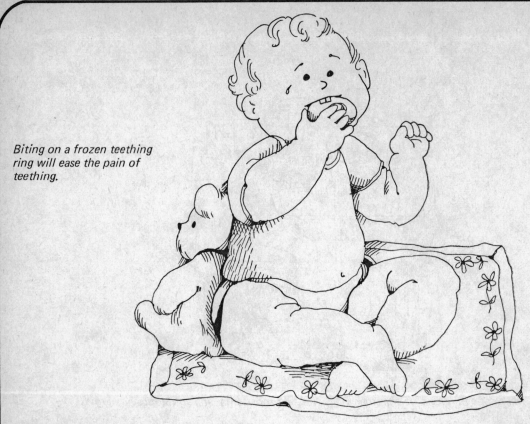

Biting on a frozen teething ring will ease the pain of teething.

Description

A baby usually will cut 20 teeth during his first three years of life. All 20 are temporary (deciduous) and are partly formed within the gums at birth. The age and sequence of the eruption of teeth varies from child to child, but usually the lower, central incisors are the first to break through the gums. (They may do so before birth or after one year of age.) The upper four incisors and the lower lateral incisors usually follow. The four one-year molars are next; then, the four canines; and finally, the four two-year molars.

Diagnosis

Teething commonly is accompanied by drooling, fretfulness, wakefulness at night, unwillingness to eat, discomfort, or chewing on fingers or objects. Drooling and chewing are not related to any abnormality; and fretfulness, wakefulness, and unwillingness to eat have a multitude of causes.

A few days before teeth erupt, they push the gum ahead of them and can be seen or felt. Before molars erupt, they frequently elicit a blue blood-blister.

Home Treatment

Teething pain may be eased by rubbing the gums, with or without anesthetics such as paregoric or commercial dental products. Biting on zwieback toast, teething biscuits, or teething rings helps the teeth erupt, and biting on cold objects (ice wrapped in cloth, frozen teething rings) numbs the gums and eases the pain of teething. Aspirin or acetaminophen also may help relieve pain, and antihistamines given at night may help the child sleep. In the daytime diversions may make the child forget the pain.

Precautions

● On and off for three years, infants will be teething. During these three years, do not blame every symptom on teething but look for other possible causes. ● Diarrhea and constipation are the result of teething only if the child alters his diet radically. ● If the child's eating and drinking habits change do not try to force-feed him. ● Fever, cough, and nasal discharge are not symptoms of teething. ● Teething may produce chapping on the face but no other rashes. ● Too liberal application of commercial teething ointments and solutions that contain local anesthetics may cause anemia.

Doctor's Treatment

Before attributing symptoms to teething, your doctor will check for other causes.

TESTICLE, TORSION OF

Description

For unknown reasons, a testicle may become twisted, shutting off the blood supply. Although the condition is more apt to affect boys with an undescended testicle, it is not rare among boys whose testes are in the normal position in the scrotum. The condition also may follow a minor injury.

Once a testicle has been twisted, it becomes slightly swollen and tender. A few hours later it is intensely painful, markedly tender, and swollen. The testicle and the skin surrounding it become discolored (red or blue), and the boy may be nauseated or vomit and have lower abdominal pain and a fever.

Diagnosis

Torsion of a testicle that has descended into the scrotum may be confused with an infection (orchitis), a strangulated hernia, or a bruise of the scrotum. Torsion of a testicle that has *not* descended and lies in the groin may be confused with a strangulated hernia, injury, or infected lymph glands in the groin. Torsion of an undescended testicle that lies within the abdominal cavity is difficult to diagnose but may be suspected whenever abdominal pain occurs. This condition represents an **emergency situation** and medical intervention should be immediate.

Torsion of a part of a testicle (appendix of the testis) causes similar, although less intense, symptoms of torsion of the entire testicle. Distinguishing between these conditions is unimportant because they are treated the same way.

Home Treatment

None. **Torsion of the testicle is a surgical emergency.**

Precautions

● Take your boy to a doctor immediately if pain near a testicle increases and the testicle is tender, swollen, or discolored. **Hours count.**
● Suspect torsion of the testicle in a boy with an uncorrected, undescended testicle if he has lower abdominal pain or pain in the groin. ● An injury or a bruise of the scrotum and testis is not uncommon and will cause instant pain that gradually subsides. If pain increases following an injury or a bruise suspect torsion of the testicle.

Doctor's Treatment

Your doctor will arrange immediate surgery to untwist the testicle and anchor it in the scrotum to prevent further episodes. If surgery is not performed within 24 hours of the onset of the symptoms the testis may be damaged permanently.

Related Topics: Hernia; Testicle, Undescended

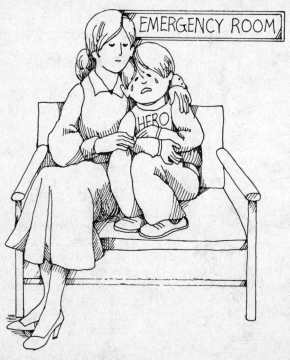

Torsion of the testicle causes intense pain and requires immediate medical attention.

TESTICLE, UNDESCENDED

Description

In the male fetus the two testicles lie just beneath the kidneys. Before birth, they migrate down into the groin and come to rest in each side of the scrotum. In one to two percent of full-term male infants and 20 to 30 percent of premature male infants the testes have not completed their descent at the time of birth. These boys have an undescended testicle.

One or both testicles may be undescended, and the undescended testis may lie within the abdomen or the groin. In a boy's first months or years of life an undescended testicle may successfully complete its migration to the scrotum. But it may not.

A testicle that remains undescended is at risk of becoming twisted, injured, or malignant. If the condition is not corrected by the time a boy reaches age seven an undescended testicle may be damaged by the heat of the body; it may shrivel (atrophy) and lose its ability to produce sperm.

Diagnosis

If one or both testicles do not rest in the scrotum at birth the infant has an undescended testicle. An undescended testicle must be distinguished from a migratory or retractile testis, however. A migrating or retractile testis has completed its descent into the scrotum, but it temporarily has risen into the groin. A migratory or retractile testis returns to its normal position as the boy matures, and it needs no correction. If the size of the scrotum is normal the testis is migrating; if it is small the testis is undescended. An undescended testicle sometimes can be felt lying along the inguinal canal, but it may be mistaken for a hernia or a swollen lymph gland.

Home Treatment

If a testicle appears to be missing from the scrotum after birth, periodically check to see if it descends of its own accord. If it does not, consult your doctor. To check for an undescended testis place the boy in a tub of warm water and pull his knees up toward his chest. If the testicle is migratory it will often descend into the scrotum. If the testicle is undescended it will not.

Precautions

● Don't worry a boy by discussing the condition. An undescended testicle usually can be corrected. ● Do not postpone correction of an undescended testicle. It should be corrected when the boy is between four and seven years old.

Doctor's Treatment

Your doctor will examine your boy's scrotum and groin carefully and check for the presence of a hernia, which often coexists with an undescended testis. Some doctors give hormone injections to encourage descent of the testicle, but most prefer to perform surgery between the ages of four and seven without using hormones.

Related Topics: Hernia; Lymph Nodes—Infection Fighters; Testicle, Torsion of

An undescended testicle should be corrected when the boy is between four and seven years old.

Description

Tetanus (lockjaw) is a disease of the nervous system that is caused by the Clostridium tetani germ. The germ grows in the absence of oxygen and normally lives in soil, dust, and the intestines and intestinal wastes of animals and humans. It easily enters the body through deep puncture wounds or lacerations, but it also may gain access to the body through a scratch, abrasion, burn, or insect bite. The germ incubates for three to twenty-one days. Once the infection is full-blown, it causes muscle stiffness, especially of the jaw and neck (giving rise to the name lockjaw); difficulty in swallowing; pain in the extremities; muscle spasms throughout the body; convulsions; and sometimes death.

Diagnosis

The diagnosis usually is evident when a child develops muscle spasms and convulsions days or weeks after sustaining a wound. However it may be confused with neonatal tetany (a generally benign condition in babies) or with a drug reaction, poisoning, meningitis, encephalitis, or rabies in older children. The diagnosis may be confirmed by isolating the Clostridium tetani germ from a wound.

Home Treatment

Prevention is the key. Be sure to take proper care of wounds, even the trivial ones, until they heal. Get your children immunized during infancy and schedule booster shots to ensure immunity for life.

Precautions

● If a new mother is not immune to tetanus her newborn baby is susceptible to tetanus. If a mother is immune her baby may be temporarily immune to it. ● In newborns the stump of the umbilical cord may be the site of tetanus' entry into the body. If a baby is delivered at home be certain to use strict antiseptic techniques during and immediately after birth. ● Be certain that all members of the family have received the initial series of tetanus toxoid immunizations and that boosters are given every ten years throughout life.

Doctor's Treatment

Your doctor will take prompt care of wounds and administer a toxoid booster to a child who has been immunized or human tetanus antiserum to one who has not. If tetanus has developed your doctor will hospitalize your child and order intensive treatment involving antiserum, antibiotics, sedation, anesthesia, and intravenous fluids. When recovered, your child should be immunized against any subsequent attack.

Related Topics: Burns, Cuts, Immunizations, Puncture Wounds, Scrapes

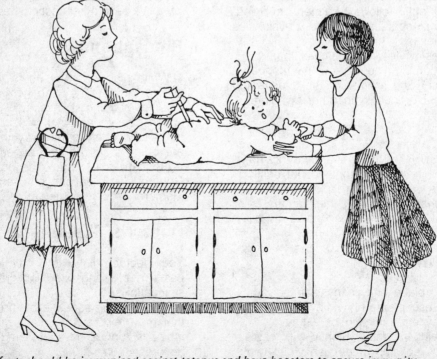

Infants should be immunized against tetanus and have boosters to ensure immunity.

THRUSH

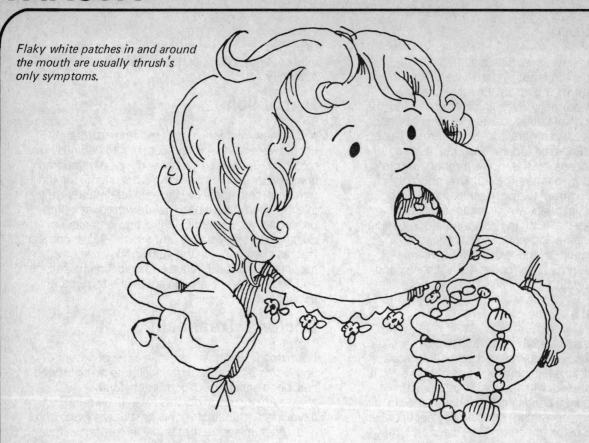

Flaky white patches in and around the mouth are usually thrush's only symptoms.

Description

Thrush is an infection of the mouth caused by the *Candida albicans* fungus. It is common in babies immediately after birth, in infants, and in toddlers. It frequently follows treatment involving antibiotics or accompanies nutritional deficiencies and chronic illnesses.

Thrush causes white, flaky patches that resemble milk curds to appear on the tongue, palate, gums, and the insides of the cheeks and lips. Generally, it produces no other symptoms.

Diagnosis

The diagnosis is based on the appearance in the mouth of white plaques that do not easily wipe away. It is confirmed by isolating the *Candida albicans* fungus from the plaques and examining them under a microscope or by a culture.

Home Treatment

To treat thrush, place one cc nystatin solution (available by prescription only) into each cheek four times a day after nursing or eating. Alternatively, paint the mouth lightly with one percent aqueous solution of gentian violet two or three times a day after nursing. Gentian violet is available without a prescription. To prevent reinfection, sterilize objects that are placed in the baby's mouth. A nursing mother may have to use nystatin cream on each breast to avoid reinfecting her baby.

Precautions

● White plaques confined to the tongue are not due to thrush. They are normally the result of nursing. ● If thrush occurs with a fever or cough see your doctor. ● If thrush recurs frequently, analyze the way the baby's things are being sterilized and consult your doctor. ● Gentian violet should be used sparingly. Generous applications or overuse can burn the membranes of the mouth.

Doctor's Treatment

Your doctor will try to determine if your child has a debilitating condition that increases his susceptibility to thrush. The child's mother may be treated for diseases of the nipples or vagina that may reinfect the infant with the *Candida albicans* fungus. Nystatin or gentian violet will be prescribed.

Description

The thyroid gland is located in the neck just below the Adam's apple; it produces hormones that control the body's metabolism rate. The thyroid gland may become underactive (hypothyroidism) or overactive (hyperthyroidism) at any age, including infancy.

Hypothyroidism. When the thyroid is underactive at birth, usually it's not apparent for a few weeks. When it finally does become apparent, it causes excessive sleepiness, choking while nursing, severe constipation, and noisy breathing. After three to six months, it is obvious that the growth rate is retarded, and the child has a protruding tongue; thick, dry skin; and a hoarse cry. When the thyroid becomes underactive later in childhood, it slows growth and causes constipation, sleepiness, and thick, dry skin. An underactive thyroid may or may not be associated with goiter.

Hyperthyroidism. An overactive thyroid usually develops between the ages of ten and fifteen, but sometimes, it may occur in children as young as age one or two years. An overactive thyroid causes irritability, restlessness, problems in school, tremors of the hands, increased appetite without weight gain, excessive sweating, and protruding eyeballs. Overactive thyroid is usually accompanied by goiter.

Diagnosis

Because all symptoms of over- and underactive thyroid can result from other conditions not related to the thyroid, laboratory tests are essential to the diagnosis. In some states, it has recently become mandatory that all newborn infants be tested for thyroid malfunction before leaving the nursery.

Home Treatment

Home care involves watching for the symptoms of a thyroid malfunction and taking your child to your doctor for routine checkups.

Precautions

● Symptoms of hypothyroidism may occur in older children, especially adolescents, who have normal thyroid function. Only your doctor can determine if the thyroid is malfunctioning. ● A child who has cysts on the neck should not have them removed until investigation shows that the cyst is not actually the thyroid gland in an abnormal position.

Doctor's Treatment

Your doctor will establish the diagnosis on the basis of a physical examination, which will include measurement of your child's blood pressure, and laboratory tests that measure thyroid and pituitary hormone levels in the blood (triiodothyronine, thyroxine, thyroid stimulating hormone). It also sometimes needs to be determined how well the thyroid absorbs radioactive iodine.

Treatment of an underactive thyroid involves oral administration of desiccated thyroid or thyroid hormones. Treatment of an overactive thyroid involves medication or surgical removal of part of the thyroid gland.

Related Topic: Goiter

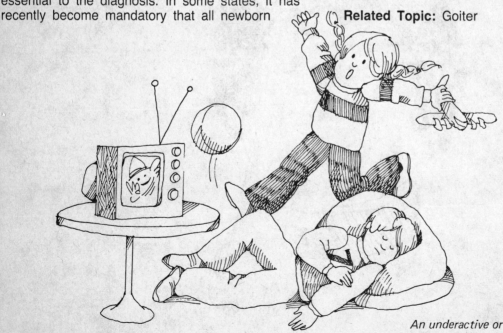

An underactive or overactive thyroid will cause changes in your child's behavior.

TICS

Description

Repetitive, jerky, spasmodic movements of isolated muscle groups are called tics. Usually, tics involve twitching the mouth, wrinkling the forehead, blinking the eyes, sighing, coughing or sniffing. The head, shoulders, hands, or arms may jerk uncontrollably. Tics may happen several times a minute or once or twice a day, and they persist for weeks or months.

Tics occur in preschool and school age children as a result of undue pressure and emotional stress. They increase when a child is upset or excited and stop temporarily when he is diverted or asleep.

A more serious but rare form of tics is Gilles de la Tourette's disease. The disease may resemble tics at the outset, but it progresses to violent twitching of the face and arms and sometimes other parts of the body. The spasmodic movements are accompanied by explosive sounds such as a barking cough or indistinct words or obscenities.

Diagnosis

Generally, tics are obvious, but they may have to be distinguished from allergies, which often lead to twitching the nose, blinking the eyes, and coughing. Gilles de la Tourette's disease is rare and progressive, and it cannot be diagnosed at the onset.

Home Treatment

Do not pay undue attention to tics. Reacting to them by calling your child's attention to them, demanding that the child stop, or berating or punishing the child may aggravate or prolong the condition. Any obvious stressful situation at home, at school, or among your child's peers should be alleviated.

Precautions

● Ignoring tics requires the cooperation of siblings, parents, relatives, neighbors, and teachers. ● If tics are the only sign of emotional tension in a child they may be due to the customary stresses of childhood. If tics persist for more than a few weeks or occur with other symptoms or patterns of disturbed emotional behavior they may signal a potentially serious problem. Seek professional advice.

Doctor's Treatment

Your doctor will rule out organic illnesses as a cause of the tic by means of a careful examination. Stressful situations in your child's environment will be evaluated and you will be advised as to how to handle them. Your doctor may require consultation with a neurologist to diagnose and treat Gilles de la Tourette's disease.

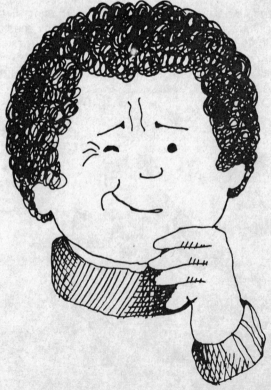

A tic is an uncontrollable twitch which may be due to stress.

TONSILLITIS

Description

The tonsils (in the throat) and the adenoids (in the back of the nose) are part of the lymphatic system, and their function is to destroy disease-causing germs. They may become mildly or chronically infected with disease-causing germs from a common cold, sore throat, mononucleosis, diphtheria, or tuberculosis.

Chronic or recurrent infections of the tonsils and adenoids can result in their permanent enlargement (hypertrophy). Enlargement of the tonsils rarely produces symptoms by itself but, in extreme cases, it may interfere with swallowing. Enlargement of the adenoids results in mouth breathing, hearing loss and middle ear infection, snoring, nasal speech, and bad breath.

A unique infection of the tonsils is Quincy sore throat (peritonsillar abscess). In Quincy a large abscess forms behind a tonsil, producing intense pain and a high fever (103°F or 104°F). The abscess eventually pushes the tonsil across the midline of the throat.

Diagnosis

Acute infection of the tonsils is diagnosed on the basis of the appearance of the throat and the results of a throat culture or blood count. Chronic infection of the adenoids and tonsils is diagnosed on the basis of frequent bouts of infection or almost constant symptoms of infection and the presence of chronically swollen lymph nodes in the neck. Enlarged tonsils can be observed in the throat, but they must not be mistaken for temporarily enlarged tonsils due to acute infection. Enlarged adenoids cannot be seen directly. Special instruments must be used or X rays may be taken.

Home Treatment

Treatment of tonsillitis is the same as treatment of the common cold, sore throat, or hay fever. A peritonsillar abscess requires treatment by a doctor.

Precautions

● Adenoids and tonsils usually are large in children three to nine years of age. Do not confuse this enlargement with one of chronic infection. ● Tonsils often contain a white, cheesy material. This material is normal; it does not indicate infection. ● Tonsils and adenoids may be chronically infected without becoming enlarged. A history of recurring infection and the condition of the lymph nodes in the neck are more reliable indicators of chronic infection than size. ● Enlarged tonsils are rarely the cause of poor eating habits.

Doctor's Treatment

Your doctor will treat a peritonsillar abscess with antibiotics; occasionally surgical drainage is necessary.

The decision to remove tonsils and adenoids surgically requires considerable evaluation. Some doctors insist that they should never be removed; others recommend routine removal. Both groups are wrong.

Tonsillectomy may be performed as part of the treatment of: a peritonsillar abscess or frequent infections (for more than a year) of the tonsils; a tonsillar tumor; or a diphtheria bacilli-infected tonsil.

Adenoidectomy may be performed to correct: a nasal obstruction which has led to facial peculiarities such as a pinched face, narrow nostrils, or constantly open mouth; a chronic cough; bad breath; snoring; or a nasal voice. It also may be wise to have adenoids removed if their enlargement is causing a hearing loss or frequent middle ear infections. Or it may be done as part of the treatment of frequent infections of the adenoids. Alternatives to adenoidectomy include prolonged use of decongestants and antibiotics or insertion of polyethylene tubes (grommets) into the ear.

Related Topics: Common Cold, Frequent Illnesses, Hay Fever, Sore Throat

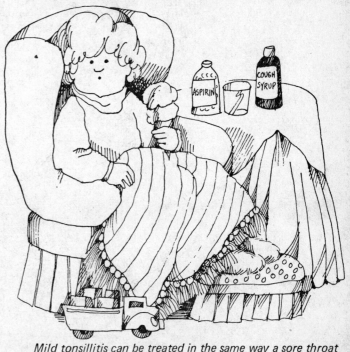

Mild tonsillitis can be treated in the same way a sore throat is treated.

TOOTHACHE

Description

In common with earaches and the onset of labor, toothaches among children begin only after druggists have closed their doors and doctors and dentists have closed their offices.

A toothache can be caused by an injury to a tooth, an infection between the gum and the tooth, or an abscess of the root of the tooth due to extension of a cavity (even a filled one) into the tooth's pulp.

Diagnosis

The source of a toothache is obvious if the gum near the tooth is red, swollen, and tender or if a cavity is visible. If the source of the pain is in doubt, tapping gently with a tongue depressor or the handle of a spoon will cause sharp pain in the tooth responsible.

Home Treatment

Temporary treatment involves the relief of pain with aspirin, acetaminophen, and/or codeine. Codeine is available in the form of cough medicine. In a pinch, cough medicines with dextromethorphan may be used for pain relief. In desperation, one teaspoon of whiskey for every 20 pounds of the child's weight—diluted with water or mixers plus sugar—will alleviate pain. An icepack on the jaw may help; but heat often will worsen a toothache. If home treatment does not relieve the toothache, a hospital emergency room should be able to furnish codeine or meperidine for that purpose.

Part of home treatment is prevention. Your child should see a dentist regularly beginning at age two or three. He should brush at least daily and use floss if possible. Through adolescence, fluoride must be provided each day. If you live in an area where the water is not fluoridated, supplementary fluoride is needed.

Precautions

● Take your child to a dentist regularly to avoid any emergency situation involving toothache.

Doctor's Treatment

Your doctor may prescribe a pain killer or an antibiotic if an infection is present. But your dentist will carry out definitive treatment.

Related Topic: Teething

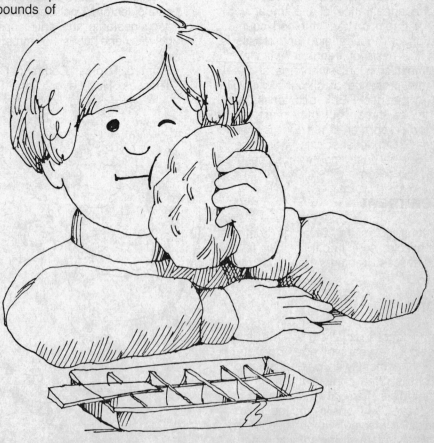

An icepack on the jaw may alleviate the pain of a toothache.

TOXOPLASMOSIS

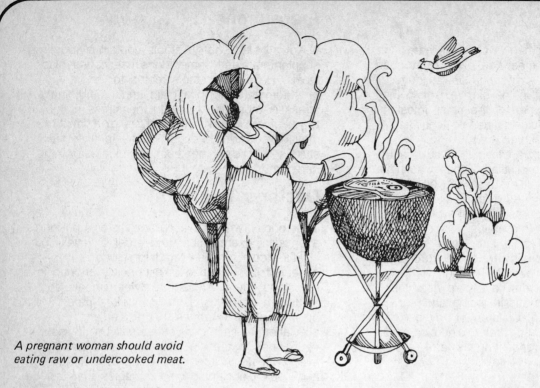

A pregnant woman should avoid eating raw or undercooked meat.

Description

Toxoplasmosis afflicts all mammals (including people), many birds, and some reptiles. It is caused by a one-celled parasite (toxoplasma) that is one-third the size of a red-blood cell. Although blood tests show that as many as half the adults in this country have had the infection at one time or another, few people outside the medical community are even aware of it. Like German measles, toxoplasmosis can severely damage the fetus during the first three months of pregnancy, but it is rarely serious for any other age group.

Most people with toxoplasmosis have no symptoms. Some have transient swelling of the lymph nodes, and a few have symptoms resembling those of infectious mononucleosis. Rarely is the illness severe. When it is, it causes a high fever (103°F or 104°F) and leads to pneumonia, encephalitis, and heart disease. One attack, however mild, seems to confer lifelong immunity.

Toxoplasmosis arises from eating raw or undercooked meat or by direct contact with the feces of chickens, cats, or dogs. The disease is not spread among humans, except from a pregnant woman to the fetus she carries.

A women who acquires toxoplasmosis during the first three months of pregnancy may transmit the infection to the fetus via the placenta. As a result, the fetus may be aborted or stillborn, or the infant may be born with water on the brain (hydrocephalus) or a pinhead (microcephaly). The newborn may have convulsions, anemia, jaundice, or eye damage.

Diagnosis

The diagnosis is usually missed. It may be suspected from a blood count that shows numerous white blood cells of a certain type, but it can be confirmed only by complicated tests that evaluate the blood levels of antibodies against toxoplasma organisms.

Home Treatment

None.

Precautions

● A pregnant woman should not expose herself to toxoplasma organisms by eating raw or undercooked meat; nor should she acquire a new pet during the first trimester of her pregnancy. However, congenital toxoplasmosis is so rare that most experienced pediatricians have never seen a case. It hardly seems necessary, therefore, for a pregnant woman to avoid eating meat altogether or to get rid of household pets.

Doctor's Treatment

Drugs are available to treat severe cases of toxoplasmosis, but they are highly toxic and cannot be given to pregnant women.

175

ULCER

Description

Ulcers are less common in children than adults, but they are by no means rare and may even occur in newborns. As with adults, children's ulcers can be found in the stomach or in the duodenum (the first part of the small intestine). (Actually, duodenal ulcers are five times more common than stomach ulcers.)

Ulcers are more common in intense, highly motivated children, particularly those who have family conflicts. But ulcers also can be precipitated by prolonged treatment with steroids, extensive burns, diseases of the brain, or severe infections (meningitis, or blood poisoning). An older child with ulcers has upper abdominal pain before meals or at night, and the pain is often relieved by eating. Preschoolers with ulcers have pain near the navel; the pain is erratic in timing and aggravated by eating. Children of any age may vomit bright red or dark brown blood or have blood in the stools (appearing as tarry stools).

Diagnosis

Although often suspected as the cause of stomach aches in children, ulcers are seldom the cause. The diagnosis of an ulcer can be made only by X rays (upper gastrointestinal series) or, less commonly, by endoscopy (direct visualization of the stomach by use of an instrument passed down the esophagus).

Home Treatment

When pain is typical of an ulcer in timing and location, temporary relief can be provided by an oral antacid. Other home treatment is not recommended.

Precautions

● Not all black (tarry) stools contain blood. Iron supplements and some foods can cause black stools. Have tarry stools tested for blood. ● Abdominal pain in a child under emotional stress is most likely due to the stress and not to an ulcer. ● Several members of a family may have ulcers because of the family's life style and tension, not because ulcers are hereditary.

Doctor's Treatment

Your doctor will take a careful history, perform a physical examination, and order X rays. Your child's stools will be tested for blood and observed for evidence of secondary anemia in the blood count. Antacids between meals and at bedtime or antispasmodics before meals will be prescribed. Changes in the diet and alleviation of emotional stress will be advised.

Changes in the diet usually involve avoiding milk; caffeine in cola drinks, tea, and coffee; and aspirin (including cold remedies that include aspirin). Treatment usually can be discontinued in a few weeks or months.

Related Topic: Stomach Ache, Chronic

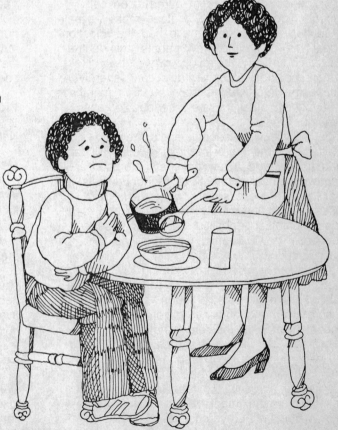

Abdominal pain before meals may signal ulcers.

URINARY TRACT INFECTION

Description

Infections of the urinary tract are common during childhood, and they are ten times more frequent in girls than in boys. About five percent of all girls will have one or more urinary tract infections before reaching maturity.

In most cases, except during infancy, no physical abnormality accounts for the development of a urinary tract infection (UTI). But for five percent of the girls and over 50 percent of the boys with UTI, an underlying anatomical abnormality somewhere along the urinary tract results in a partial or total block in the flow of urine. Most UTIs are caused by germs, such as E. coli bacilli, that do not cause disease in other locations. E. coli bacilli live peacefully in the bowels of all children and adults but cause infection when they ascend the urethra (the tube that leads to the urinary bladder). Other causes of UTI are inflammation of the vagina, foreign bodies in the bladder or urethra, and possibly severe constipation.

The urinary tract is a series of interconnected tubes; an infection in one part easily spreads to another. For this reason, this discussion does not distinguish among infection of the collecting basins of the kidneys (pyelonephritis and pyelitis), infection of the tubes that connect the kidneys to the bladder (ureteritis), infection of the bladder (cystitis), and infection of the urethra (urethritis).

A urinary tract infection may elicit no symptoms at all (silent UTI) or any combination of the following: urgency, frequency, or pain on urination; dribbling of urine; bedwetting; daytime incontinence; foul-smelling, cloudy, or bloody urine; fever; abdominal or back pain; vomiting; and redness of the external genitalia. If the infection goes untreated, the symptoms generally disappear in a few days or weeks and often return later.

Diagnosis

The diagnosis of UTI depends upon a careful physical examination and urinalysis and urine culture. In boys, the diagnosis involves a search for an obstruction in the urinary tract. In girls, the search for an obstruction is undertaken only after two or three bouts of UTI or one bout with an infection that is resistant to treatment. In infants, investigation for the underlying cause is always undertaken immediately.

Home Treatment

Any attempt at home is potentially dangerous and may result in a low-grade, destructive infection with no outward symptoms.

Precautions

● Fever, but few or no other symptoms, and a normal physical examination are a common UTI profile, particularly if it is a recurrent pattern.
● To obtain a urine specimen for analysis or culture, cleanse the genitalia and collect the portion at the midpoint of urination. In this way, the urine sample will not be contaminated.

Doctor's Treatment

Your doctor will conduct a complete physical examination including measurement of your child's blood pressure, urinalysis and urine culture. Appropriate antibiotics will be prescribed for ten to fourteen days. Urine samples will be tested during and after the course of antibiotics.

After your child has recovered from a UTI infection, your doctor may recommend X rays to rule out a physical abnormality. Sometimes, further X rays and direct examination of urethra and bladder are necessary. To treat recurrent UTIs that are not due to obstruction, your doctor may prescribe the use of antibiotics—constantly or intermittently for months or years. To correct an obstruction, your doctor will perform surgery.

Related Topic: Bedwetting

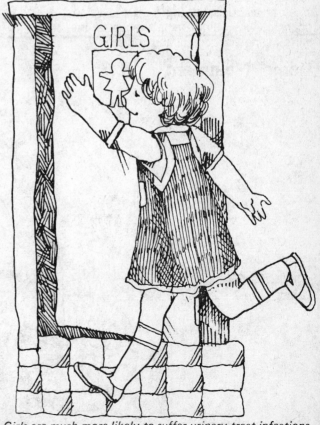

Girls are much more likely to suffer urinary tract infections than are boys.

VAGINAL BLEEDING

Description

Bloody vaginal discharge may occur during the first two weeks of a girl's life, and it is usually due to her mother's hormones. But the most common cause of vaginal bleeding is, of course, menstruation, which may begin any time between the ages of nine and seventeen. So-called precocious puberty may begin before age nine, even as early as five or six. With menstruation and precocious puberty, the first menstrual flow is preceded by breast development.

Vaginal bleeding any time after the neonatal period (in a girl without breast development) or bleeding between menstrual periods is most often due to injury. Wounds in the vaginal area, even those of considerable size, heal rapidly with no infection or scarring.

Less common causes of vaginal bleeding are inflammation of the vagina, a foreign body in the vagina, prolapse of the lining of the urethra (the tube leading to the urinary bladder), and tumors of the vagina or the uterus.

Diagnosis

Diagnosis of the cause of abnormal vaginal bleeding often can be made by inspecting the vaginal area. The inspection should determine whether blood is issuing from the vaginal opening, the urethra, a laceration of the surrounding tissues, or the rectum.

Home Treatment

Unless they are extensive or may be due to sexual molestation, bruises and lacerations of the vagina and the surrounding area usually can be treated at home. No antiseptic is necessary, and burning on urination can be minimized by applying an anesthetic ointment to the area or having the child urinate while in a bathtub of water. All other causes of vaginal bleeding require your doctor's attention.

Precautions

● Girls whose mothers received diethylstilbesterol (DES) during pregnancy may have a deformity of the vagina (adenosis) that causes bleeding. Whether or not they have vaginal bleeding, all girls whose mothers took DES should be examined by an experienced gynecologist at the beginning of puberty. Although the probability of malignancy associated with this drug originally was overestimated, a malignancy is still possible, and all girls with adenosis of the vagina should be carefully monitored.

Doctor's Treatment

Your doctor will determine what is causing vaginal bleeding by performing a careful examination, sometimes involving the rectum. Your doctor may require a culture of any vaginal discharge or may require an X ray of the pelvis. A girl whose mother received DES will be referred to a gynecologist. Treatment of vaginal bleeding depends upon its cause, but a prolapsed urethra requires surgical correction.

Related Topic: Vaginal Discharge

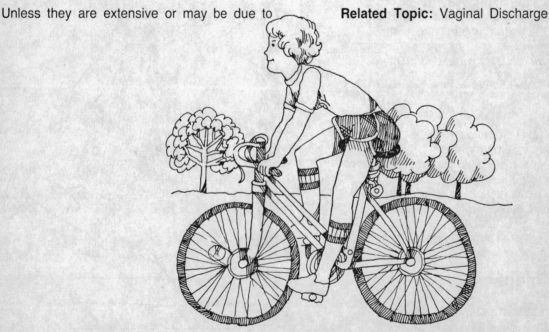

Menstruation, the most common cause of vaginal bleeding, should not curtail a girl's activities.

VAGINAL DISCHARGE

Description

Mucus discharge from the vagina is normal during the first two weeks of a girl's life and during the one to two years preceding menstruation. Such vaginal discharge may be quite profuse but it is not malodorous or irritating to the skin.

Vaginal discharge that irritates nearby membranes, smells foul, and causes itching, soreness, or pain may be caused by using chemicals in the bath (bubble bath, water softeners) or vaginal hygiene sprays, wearing panties made from synthetic materials, or improper toileting. It may be the result of pinworms or a urinary tract infection, or it may be due to masturbation, foreign bodies in the vagina, or a lack of cleanliness. In addition, vaginal discharge may arise from vaginal infection (vaginitis) due to viral or bacterial microorganisms (coliform bacilli, streptococci, staphylococci, pneumococci, gonococci, or herpes) or yeasts.

Diagnosis

Vaginal discharge that occurs during puberty and is not irritating or malodorous is normal. Vaginal discharge that is pus-like, irritating, foul smelling, or bloody is abnormal. But the cause of the problem usually must be determined by your doctor.

Home Treatment

Some of the simple causes of abnormal vaginal discharges can be eliminated. Avoid using vaginal sprays and chemicals in bath water, buy cotton underpants, and instruct your daughter to wipe herself from front to back after going to the bathroom. Look for signs of pinworms or urinary tract infections. Bland ointments such as A and D or Desitin rash remedies or petroleum jelly may be helpful and so may taking sitz baths in a tub of water to which a cup of vinegar has been added.

Precautions

- Girls whose mothers received diethylstibesterol (DES) while pregnant may have a deformity of the vagina (adenosis) that causes vaginal discharge. Such girls should be examined by a gynecologist whether or not they have vaginal discharge.

Doctor's Treatment

Your doctor will take a detailed history and conduct a physical (including rectal) examination. A culture and a smear of the discharge and sometimes an X ray of the pelvis will be taken. Your doctor may also order urinanalysis and urine culture.

Treatment depends upon the cause of the problem, but it may involve the use of antibiotics, worm medicine, fungicides, medicated suppositories, or hormone ointments.

Related Topics: Pinworms, Urinary Tract Infection, Vaginal Bleeding

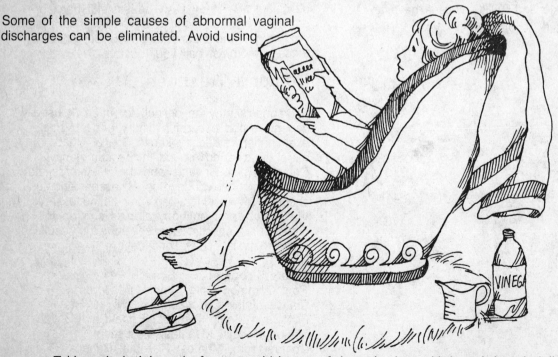

Taking a sitz bath in a tub of water to which a cup of vinegar has been added may help vaginal discharge.

VIRUSES

Description

A virus is a germ that is smaller than a bacterium, and can live only within a living cell. Many common illnesses are caused by a particular virus: mumps, chicken pox, measles, rubella, mononucleosis, cat scratch fever, hepatitis, warts, molluscum, and roseola. And two large groups of other viruses cause a variety of similar illnesses in children: the respiratory viruses and the intestinal viruses.

The respiratory viruses include the adenoviruses, parainfluenza viruses, the rhinoviruses, influenza viruses and the respiratory syncytial virus. The *intestinal viruses* (enteroviruses) inhabit the intestinal tract and are divided into Coxsackie viruses (of which 30 varieties are known so far), enteric cytopathogenic human orphan (ECHO) virus (with 31 known types), and the three polio viruses. Coxsackie viruses are responsible for hand, foot, and mouth disease, herpangina, and pleurodynia. Herpangina lasts three to six days and produces a fever, sore throat, swollen neck glands, and painful ulcers on the soft palate, tonsils, and throat. Pleurodynia is an inflammation of the nerves between the ribs, and it causes intense pain on one side of the chest, which is aggravated by breathing.

ECHO viruses may cause diarrhea. And Coxsackie and ECHO viruses may cause symptoms of a common cold, a fever with or without a rash, encephalitis, or paralysis.

The Coxsackie and ECHO viruses have an incubation period of three to five days or more,

and they can be spread via the oral or the fecal route. Immunity against any one of them is short lived. Therefore, a child can have one virus right after another.

Diagnosis

Because of the large number of viruses and the multiplicity of symptoms, diagnosis is very difficult. Herpangina usually can be identified by the look and location of the ulcers. Pleurodynia resembles pleurisy and pneumonia, but it produces no cough. A rash due to a virus tends to be generalized, flat, and pink rather than red and splotchy, but rashes vary considerably from child to child.

Home Treatment

Only the symptoms of illnesses caused by intestinal viruses can be treated. To reduce pain and fever, give aspirin or acetaminophen. To relieve severe pain from pleurodynia or herpangina, try codeine.

Precautions

● Coxsackie and ECHO viruses do NOT cause the following symptoms: a rash that looks like red sandpaper or red goosebumps; pus-like discharge from the eyes, nose, or ears; reddish-purple spots; tender, red lymph nodes that continue to enlarge; severe earaches; blood in the stools; severe cough; or breathing difficulties. But they CAN cause: stiff neck or back; severe headache and vomiting; paralysis; prostration; and disorientation. If your child has these symptoms, call your doctor.

Doctor's Treatment

A diagnosis may be difficult to reach. It usually depends upon a careful history and physical examination, aided by knowledge of what currently is going around in the community. Complete blood counts and throat cultures may be needed to exclude other illnesses, and a chest X ray or spinal tap may be necessary. Viral cultures or antibody studies confirm the presence of specific diseases, but the results of these tests take days or weeks.

Related Topics: Cat Scratch Fever; Chicken Pox; Common Cold; Diarrhea/Children; Diarrhea/Infants; Encephalitis; Fever; Hand, Foot, and Mouth Disease; Hepatitis; Infectious Mononucleosis; Measles; Molluscum Contagiosum; Mumps; Roseola; Rubella; Glands, Swollen; Ulcers; Warts

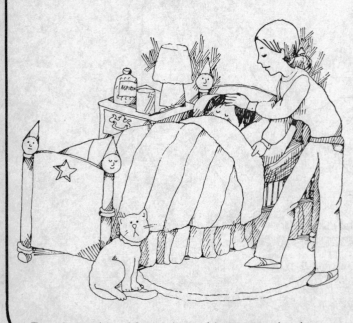

To reduce pain and fever, give aspirin or acetaminophen.

Description

At birth, a baby who has normal eyes cannot focus on an object or visually follow movement. If an infant's eyes seem to make random, searching movements, he may have defective vision. By age four or five, five to ten percent of all children have a visual problem. By the end of adolescence, the percentage has climbed to thirty.

The usual visual problems among children and adolescents are nearsightedness (myopia), amblyopia ex anopsia (lazy eye), farsightedness (hyperopia), and astigmatism. Nearsightedness, or the inability to see distant objects clearly, is hereditary. It is rarely present at birth but increases as the child grows. Amblyopia develops during the first six or seven years of life. Farsightedness (inability to see nearby objects clearly) and astigmatism (blurred vision at all distances) occur at an early age and don't usually grow worse with time.

There are clear symptoms that may indicate poor vision. If your child habitually tilts his head or looks out of the corner of his eyes; if his eyes cross or deviate from normal, he squints, or is excessively sensitive to bright lights, there could be an eyesight problem. Holding objects close to examine them, failure to recognize familiar people at a distance, headaches following use of the eyes, problems in school, and a dislike of reading may also signify poor vision.

Diagnosis

Vision can be tested at different ages in a variety of ways. During the first week of life an infant should fix his eyes on a bright light. By two months of age, his eyes should follow that light as it moves through a 180-degree arc. By seven or eight months the infant should be able to recognize and respond to facial expressions. After age three, a child's eyes can be tested by having him focus on charts that use pictures or the letter E pointed in different directions. Finally, around age five or six, the child's eyes can be tested using a standard Snellen eye chart. An ophthalmologist can estimate the visual sharpness of even very young children under general anesthesia if necessary.

Home Treatment

Be alert to the symptoms that indicate impaired vision and have the child's eyes periodically examined.

Precautions

● If a child cannot see the television screen from a distance or holds books close to his eyes he may be nearsighted. ● A child's vision should be checked annually, beginning no later than age four.

Doctor's Treatment

At each annual eye checkup, your doctor will examine the exterior and interior of your child's eyes with an ophthalmoscope and test his vision using a chart of letters in rows of diminishing sizes. If an abnormality is suspected, your doctor will refer your child to an eye specialist for more detailed examination and correction of the problem.

Related Topics: Crossed Eyes, Lazy Eye

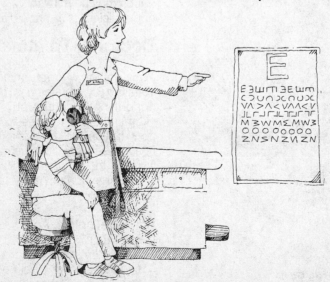

All children should have their vision tested periodically.

VOMITING

Description

Vomiting is a common occurrence during childhood. In most instances, it is merely a nuisance, but at times it can hinder the work of medications or promote dehydration through the loss of fluids.

Most infants spit up and occasionally vomit. If vomiting does not hinder weight gain, it is neither harmful nor abnormal. Excessive vomiting, however, may indicate an intolerance of formula, milk, or some foods. Frequent, forceful vomiting during an infant's first month suggests an obstruction at the end of the stomach (pylorospasm or pyloric stenosis).

In children, a viral infection of the digestive tract (gastroenteritis or intestinal flu) or an infectious disease elsewhere in the body can cause vomiting. Less common causes are abnormalities of the brain (concussion, migraine, meningitis, encephalitis, tumors); poisoning; appendicitis; severe emotional distress; jaundice; foreign bodies in the digestive tract; abdominal injuries; and motion sickness.

Diagnosis

The diagnosis is determined by identifying the reason for the vomiting. Another important factor is evaluating the degree of dehydration caused by persistent vomiting.

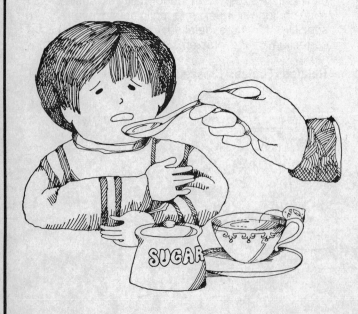

When your child is vomiting, you can give him sips of sugared tea or cold, clear liquids.

Home Treatment

When your child is vomiting, do not give him solid foods, milk, or oral aspirin; they aggravate vomiting. Aspirin may be given by rectal suppository if necessary. Do allow him sips of cold, clear liquids (ice chips, carbonated beverages, tea with sugar, liquid gelatin dessert, water, Pedialyte or Lytren—mineral and electrolyte solutions—or apple juice are good). Commercial preparations of orthophosphoric acid, fructose, and glucose also may be given. If a teaspoon of liquid is retained every five minutes, two ounces of fluid will be retained in an hour.

Some physicians warn against the use of antiemetic medications because they may obscure the diagnosis and possibly provoke Reye's syndrome (characterized by swelling of the brain and enlargement of the liver). However, dimenhydrinate in liquid or tablet form is recommended by thousands of practicing physicians, and it has effectively prevented dehydration in many children. (The drug is most effective if nothing is taken by mouth for at least an hour after the first dose. The drug should be repeated every four hours.)

Precautions

● Watch for signs of dehydration in your child.
● Medication to relieve diarrhea often aggravates vomiting. If vomiting and diarrhea are happening simultaneously treat the vomiting until it stops; then treat the diarrhea.
● Some phenothiazines that are used to stop vomiting in adults may cause serious central nervous system side effects in children; do not use them for children. Remember that abdominal pain (with or without vomiting) is appendicitis until proved otherwise.

Doctor's Treatment

Your doctor will determine the cause of vomiting by obtaining a detailed history and performing a careful physical and neurological examination. The presence and degree of dehydration will be assessed and your child hospitalized for administration of intravenous fluids if the condition is serious. Chlorpromazine or dimenhydrinate may be prescribed to relieve vomiting.

Related Topics: Appendicitis; Concussion; Dehydration; Diarrhea; Encephalitis; Gastroenteritis, Acute; Headaches; Jaundice; Meningitis; Motion Sickness; Poisoning; Stomach Ache, Acute; Stomach Ache, Chronic; Viruses

Description

A wart is a growth on the skin caused by a specific virus. Although warts may differ in appearance, they are caused by the same virus. The *common wart* is an ordinary, rough, raised wart that ranges in size from one-eighth to one inch and occurs anywhere on the skin. A *juvenile wart* is a small (one-sixteenth to one-fourth inch), smooth, pinkish wart that is common on the hands. Warts on the soles of the feet are *plantar warts.* They may be pressed into the foot (sometimes to a depth of a quarter inch or more) and often are surrounded by a callus. Groups of plantar warts are known as "mosaic warts."

Warts can be spread by direct contact or by scratching. Plantar warts can be contracted by walking barefooted where someone who has them recently walked.

For 67 percent of the children who have them, warts disappear on their own within two or three years; and for 95 percent of the children, warts will be gone within ten years. Still, some warts must be treated. Plantar warts usually require treatment because they cause pain. Warts that extend under the nails may produce permanent deformities if they are not treated. And warts on the face and eyelids are removed for cosmetic reasons. All other warts are harmless and can be ignored unless they are annoying, bleed frequently, or become infected.

Diagnosis

Many warts are unmistakable, but some are not. If in doubt, scrape or cut off the surface of the wart. If the growth is a wart, you will see pinpoint bleeding. When they are tiny, plantar warts may be mistaken for small brown splinters on the sole of the foot. They also may be indistinguishable when surrounded by a callus.

Home Treatment

To safely remove warts (other than those on the face) use Whitfield's ointment; five percent to ten percent benzoyl peroxide ointment; 40 percent salicylic acid plasters; vitamin A acid ointment; a gelatinous salicylic acid and lactic acid; or one of several commercial wart preparations such as Compound W or Vergo wart removers. Usually, treatment must continue for many days or weeks.

Precautions

• Do not treat any warts on the face or eyelids at home. • If excessive pain or redness occurs on the surrounding skin, stop treatment.
• Plantar warts may be removed by home treatment, but the success rate is small.
• Warts that involve the cuticles or extend under the nails should not be treated at home.

Doctor's Treatment

No treatment is successful in all cases. Treatment may even spread warts, or they may recur following treatment. In general, your doctor will remove warts with acids, podophyllin, electric cauterization, surgery (curetting), liquid nitrogen, solid carbon dioxide, or phenol.

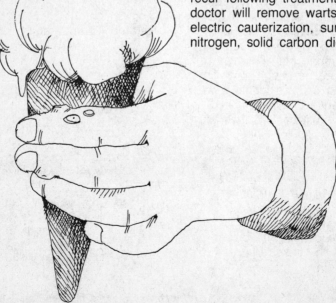

Over-the-counter preparations will safely remove warts, but treatment must continue for many days or weeks.

WHOOPING COUGH

Description

Whooping cough is the most misunderstood childhood illness today. It is a highly contagious infection of the respiratory tract, usually caused by Bordetella pertussis, but sometimes caused by Bordetella parapertussis or Bordetella bronchiseptica. Whooping cough caused by one organism does NOT provide immunity against whooping cough caused by other germs, and the vaccine provides immunity only against infection from Bordetella pertussis. The incubation period is seven to fourteen days.

In an unimmunized individual, whooping cough begins with a runny noise, low-grade fever (100°F, orally or 101°F, rectally) and a cough that gradually worsens over the next two to three weeks. Then, the cough becomes characteristic: It is worse at night than during the day and paroxysmal (several coughs occur at once without inhalation in between). At the end of a spasm the child makes a "whoop" or strangling sound as air is sucked into the lungs; vomiting of thick mucus follows. The severe, strangling cough persists for another two to three weeks and gradually subsides in three to six more weeks. But the cough may return with new respiratory infections.

Whooping cough can be serious in infants under one year. As many as 50 percent of these infants die. Newborns are not immune,

Diagnosis

In an unimmunized child, the diagnosis is unmistakable as whooping cough runs its course. The diagnosis may not be obvious, however, in infants who never develop a "whoop."

In an immunized child, the diagnosis may be impossible. The child who has been immunized may have full or partial immunity, but without boosters the immunity declines over the years. A child who is partially immune may have a mild (aborted) case of whooping cough that produces none of whooping cough's identifiable characteristics. In the absence of characteristic symptoms laboratory tests must confirm the diagnosis for most diseases. But for whooping cough, laboratory tests are to no avail. All the organisms that cause whooping cough are difficult to grow on cultures and more modern techniques for the isolation of these organisms are not readily available. Because it may be difficult to diagnose and both doctors and parents hold the misconception that the disease is rare, over 90 percent of the cases of whooping cough are not detected or even suspected.

Home Treatment

Cough suppressants may help, but no cough mixture is very effective. A child who has whooping cough should be isolated from young siblings. He should receive several small feedings a day when vomiting is severe.

Precautions

● Infants should be immunized against whooping cough. They are not naturally immune to the disease, and the mortality rate among infants with whooping cough is high. ● A child who has a mild cough might have aborted whooping cough and could spread the disease. Avoid unnecessary exposure to others. ● If your child has been exposed to whooping cough take him to a doctor. ● Whooping cough abounds, particularly in adolescents and young adults whose immunity has weakened; report to a doctor any cough that is getting progressively worse at the end of two weeks.

Doctor's Treatment

Your doctor will try to establish a diagnosis with the help of a complete blood count and cultures of the nose and throat. Most often, however, the patient's history and the doctor's clinical judgment are all that are dependable. Your doctor may prescribe erythromycin for ten to fourteen days to counter contagiousness. If given early enough, it may shorten the course of the illness. Oral steroids will lessen the severity of the cough. If your child has been exposed to whooping cough, he may receive oral erythromycin, a booster shot of vaccine, or a large dose of human antipertussis serum.

Related Topic: Immunizations

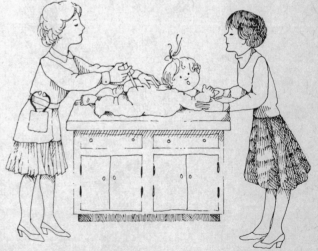

Infants, who are not naturally immune to whooping cough, should be immunized by a doctor against this potentially deadly disease.

INDEX

cracking between the toes,
  in athlete's foot, 28
cradle cap, 57
cramps,
  with diarrhea in infants, 68
  with gastroenteritis, acute, 91
Crede treatment,
  for gonorrhea, 95
creeping eruption, 58
Crohn's disease, 67
cromolyn sodium,
  for hay fever, 100
crossed eyes, 59
crotonyl-N-ethyl-o-toluide,
  for scabies, 148
croup, 15, 60, 88
  and shortness of breath, 153
  types of, 60
curvature of the spine, 150
  with backaches, 29
cutaneous larvae migrans, see
  creeping eruption
cuts, 61
cyanosis,
  with bronchiolitis, 39
cystic fibrosis, 62, 88
cystitis,
  and pinworms, 136
cysts, 22
  versus styes, 162
cytosine arabinoside,
  for herpes simplex, 106

D

deafness, 63
  and mumps, 130
  and rubella, 147
  and speech problems, 157
Debrox ear drops,
  for wax removal, 63
decongestants, 15
  for hay fever, 100
  for hives, 108
  for nosebleeds, 133
  for sinusitis, 154
deformity,
  with sprains and dislocations, 158
dehydration, 64
  and shortness of breath, 153
  with diabetes, 65
  with diarrhea, 67
  with diarrhea in infants, 68
  with gastroenteritis, acute, 91
Desitin ointment,
  for diaper rash, 66
  for vaginal discharge, 179
dexamethasone,
  for hay fever, 100
dextro-amphetamine,
  for hyperactivity, 110
dextromethorphan,
  for toothache, 174
diabetes, 65
  and shortness of breath, 153
diaper rashes, 66
diarrhea, 67
  in appendicitis, 25
  in botulism, 36
  in dysentery, 74
  in food poisoning, 85
  in infants, 68
  in influenza, 114
  in intestinal allergies, 117
  in stomach ache, chronic, 160
diarrhea, chronic
  and teething, 166

in anemia, 23
in cystic fibrosis, 62
in gastroenteritis, acute, 91
dilated pupils,
  in botulism, 36
dimenhydrinate, 14
  for dizziness, 72
  for motion sickness, 129
diminished hearing,
  with earache, 75
diphenoxylate,
  for diarrhea, 67
diphtheria, 16, 60, 69
diphtheria antitoxin, 69
diphtheria, tetanus, whooping cough
  vaccine, 16
discharge from ear, 73
  in swimmer's ear, 165
discharge from penis,
  in gonorrhea, 95
diseases requiring immunizations, 16-17
dislocations, 158
  elbow, 70
  hip, 71
disorientation,
  in encephalitis, 78
dizziness, 72
  with fainting, 82
double vision,
  in botulism, 36
draining ear, 73
  as a complication of earache, 75
Dramamine,
  for appendicitis, 25
drooling,
  with teething, 166
drowsiness,
  in concussion, 44
  in dehydration, 64
dryness of the mouth,
  in dehydration, 64
dry skin,
  and hypothyroidism, 171
DTP vaccine, see diphtheria, tetanus,
  and whooping cough vaccine
dysentery, 74, 85
  versus diarrhea, 74

E

earaches, 14, 19, 75
  in common colds, 50
  in hay fever, 100
ear canal problems, 63
eardrum and middle ear problems, 63
eardrum, rupture,
  and draining ear, 73
ear infections, 17, 19, 76
ear injury, 75
earplugs,
  for swimmer's ear, 165
earring problems, 76
earwax, impacted, 75
ECHO viruses, 180
eczema, 77
  of the ear, 76
  with intestinal allergies, 117
eighth cranial nerve problems, 63
elbow, anatomy discussed, 70
elbow, dislocated, 70
elevated blood sugar,
  in diabetes, 65
emetic, 14
Emetrol,
  for appendicitis, 25
emotional outburst,
  in hyperactivity, 110

emotional stress,
  with stomach ache, chronic, 160
emotions,
  and asthma, 27
encephalitis, 17, 78, 180
  and chicken pox, 45
  and dizziness, 72
  and measles, 124
  and toxoplasmosis, 175
enema,
  for appendicitis, 25
  for constipation, 53
enteric cytopathogenic human orphan
  (ECHO) viruses, 180
enteroviruses, 180
enuresis, see bedwetting
ephedrine,
  for asthma, 27
  for eye allergies, 79
epiglottitis, 60
  and shortness of breath, 153
epilepsy, see convulsions without fever
epinephrine,
  for insect bites, 116
Epsom salt solution,
  for blisters, 33
  for blood poisoning, 34
  for boils, 35
  for earlobe infection, 75
  for puncture wounds, 142
erythema infectiosom, 83
erythema multiforme, 108
erythroblastosis fetalis, 119
erythromycin,
  for diphtheria, 69
  for whooping cough, 184
Escherichia coli bacillus, 177
esotropia, 59
ethyl chloride,
  for creeping eruption, 58
exotropia, 59
expectorant cough remedy
  for laryngitis, 121
eye allergies, 14, 79
eye drops, antibiotic,
  for styes, 162
eye injuries, 80
eyes not parallel,
  in concussion, 51
eye tearing, 81

F

failure to thrive,
  in intestinal allergies, 117
fainting, 82
farsightedness, 181
  and lazy eye, 122
fatigue,
  with diabetes, 65
  with hay fever, 100
  with influenza, 114
  with pneumonia, 138
femoral anteversion, 135
femoral hernia, 105
femoral torsion, 135
fever, 12-13, 14, 19
  treatment of, 13
  with appendicitis, 25
  with arthritis, 26
  with blood poisoning, 34
  with bronchiolitis, 39
  with bronchitis, 40
  with cat scratch fever, 43
  with chest pain, 44
  with chicken pox, 45
  with common colds, 50

itching,
  with athlete's foot, 28
  with eczema, 77
  with eye allergies, 79
  with hand, foot, and mouth disease, 99
  with hay fever, 100
  with head lice infestation, 101
  with heat rash, 103
  with hives, 108
  with pinworms, 136
  with poison ivy, 139
  with scabies, 148
  with vaginal discharge, 179

J

Jacksonian seizures,
  in convulsions without fever, 55
jaundice, 118, 119
  in children, 118
  in newborns, 119
  with anemia, 23
  with hepatitis, 104
joint, stiff,
  with arthritis, 26
joint, swollen,
  with arthritis, 26
joint, tender,
  with arthritis, 26
  with pityriasis rosea, 137
juvenile wart, 183

K

Kaolin,
  for diarrhea, 67
  for diarrhea in infants, 68
knee, anatomy described, 120
knee pains, 120
Koplik's spots, 124

L

lacerations (cuts), 142
  of vagina, 178
lack of concentration,
  in hyperactivity, 110
lactase deficiency,
  with stomach ache, chronic, 160
lactic acid,
  for warts, 183
laryngitis, 121
larynx abnormalities,
  with speech problems, 157
laxative, 19
  for appendicitis, 25
lazy eye, 59, 122, 181
learning disabilities,
  in hyperactivity, 110
Legg-Calve-Perthes disease, 107
lethargy,
  with pityriasis rosea, 137
  with shingles, 152
leukemia, 12, 93, 123
life style,
  and ulcers, 176
lightheadedness,
  with fainting, 82
lindane,
  for head lice, 101
  for scabies, 148
lip abnormalities,
  with speech problems, 157
liver enlargement, 123
lockjaw, see tetanus
loss of consciousness, see fainting
loss of elasticity of the skin,
  in dehydration, 64

loss of function,
  with sprains and dislocations, 158
low blood sugar,
  with fainting, 82
lubricant, 15
lymph nodes, 20-21
  anterior cervical, 20
  axillary, 20
  diagnostic significance of, 21
  epitrochlear, 20
  femoral, 20
  function of, 20
  inguinal, 20
  occipital, 20
  postauricular, 20
  posterior cervical, 20
  preauricular, 20
lymph node, enlargement, 93
  with blood poisoning, 34
  with cat scratch fever, 43
  with common cold, 50
  with diphtheria, 69
  with earache, 75
  with head lice infestation, 101
  with infectious mononucleosis, 113
  with leukemia, 123
  with roseola, 146
  with rubella, 147
  with shingles, 152
  with strep throat, 161
  with swimmer's ear, 165
  with tonsillitis, 173
  with toxoplasmosis, 175
  with viral infection, 80
lymphocytes, 20
Lytren,
  for dehydration, 64

M

malaise,
  with bronchitis, 40
  with infectious mononucleosis, 113
  with polio, 141
Malgaigne's subluxation, 70
mastoiditis,
  as a complication of earaches, 75
measles, 124
  and nightmares, 132
measles, mumps, rubella vaccine, 17
mebendazole,
  for pinworms, 136
medications, 18-19
  dosage, 18
  duration of, 19
  for infants, 19
  for older children, 19
  methods of administration, 19
  rectal, 19
  timing, 18
medicine chest, pediatric, 14
  recommended contents, 14
memory loss,
  with concussion, 51
menarche, 126
Meniere's syndrome,
  and dizziness, 72
meningitis, 125
  and dizziness, 72
  as a complication of earache, 75
  in dysentery, 74
meningococci vaccine, 17
meningococcus, 125
menstruation, 126
menstruation, excessive,
  with anemia, 23
mental retardation,

and reading difficulties, 143
  and speech problems, 157
meperidine, 174
merthiolate antiseptic,
  for puncture wounds, 142
metaproterenol,
  for asthma, 27
methylphenidate,
  for hyperactivity, 110
middle ear infection,
  and draining ear, 73
  and strep throat, 161
miliaria, see heat rash
mineral oil,
  for constipation, 53
minimal brain dysfunction, 110
MMR vaccine, see measles, mumps, rubella vaccine
moles, 127
molluscum contagiosum, 128
mononucleosis, infectious, 93
motion sickness, 129
mumps, 130
muscle aches,
  with influenza, 114
  with polio, 141
muscle spasms,
  with asthma, 27
  with tetanus, 169
muscle strains,
  with chest pain, 44
muscle weakness,
  and scoliosis, 150
mycoplasma, 39
mycoplasmal pneumonia, 138
myelitis, 141
myopia, 181

N

narrowing of visual fields,
  with fainting, 82
nasal aspirator, 15
nasal congestion,
  with bronchiolitis, 39
  with bronchitis, 40
  with common colds, 50
  with hay fever, 100
nasal discharge,
  with bronchitis, 40
  with common colds, 50
  with hay fever, 100
nausea, 14
  with botulism, 36
  with fainting, 82
  with fifth disease, 83
  with hepatitis, 104
  with motion sickness, 129
  with polio, 141
  with torsion of testicle, 167
nearsightedness, 181
nephritis, 131
  and strep throat, 161
nightmares, 132
nodding of head,
  in convulsions without fever, 55
nose abnormalities,
  with speech problems, 157
nosebleeds, 133
  in leukemia, 123
nose drops, 15
nose infection,
  in diphtheria, 69
nursemaid's elbow, 70
nystatin,
  for thrush, 170

O

opiates,
opium, tincture of,
  for diarrhea in infants, 68
orchitis, 167
orthopedic shoes,
  for flat feet, 84
Osgood-Schlatter's disease, 120
OTC over-the-counter medications, 19

P

pain
  with acute synovitis of the hip, 107
  with backaches, 29
  with boils, 35
  with conjunctivitis, 52
  with dislocated elbow, 70
  with earache, 75
  with fainting, 82
  with fractures, 86
  with gum boils, 97
  with hip problems, 107
  with ingrown toenails, 115
  with Legg-Calve-Perthes disease, 107
  with pityriasis rosea, 137
  with shingles, 152
  with sinusitis, 154
  with slipped femoral epiphysis, 107
  with sore heels, 155
  with styes, 162
  with swimmer's ear, 165
  with tonsillitis, 173
  with toothache, 174
  with vaginal discharge, 179
paleness,
  in leukemia, 123
pancreatic enzymes,
  for cystic fibrosis, 62
parainfluenza viruses, 39, 60, 180
paralysis, 180
  in polio, 141
paraphimosis, 48
paregoric,
  for appendicitis, 25
  for diarrhea, 67
parent/physician partnership, 10-11
patches, crusted,
  in cradle cap, 57
patches, scaly,
  in cradle cap, 57
  in pityriasis rosea, 137
patches, yellowish,
  in cradle cap, 57
pectin,
  for diarrhea, 67, 68
Pedialyte,
  for dehydration, 64
pediatrician, how to choose, 10-11
pediatric medicine chest, 14
pemoline,
  for hyperactivity, 110
penicillin,
  for diphtheria, 69
  for impetigo, 112
  for meningitis, 125
  for strep throat, 161
perforated ear,
  as a complication of earache, 75
perforation of intestines,
  with dysentery, 74
peritonsillar abscess, 173
perleche, 134
pertussis, see whooping cough
petechiae, 41
  with gastroenteritis, acute, 91
  with meningitis, 125

petit mal, see convulsions without fever
petroleum jelly,
  for burns, 42
  for diaper rash, 66
  for nosebleeds, 133
phenylephrine,
  for eye allergies, 79
phimosis, 48
physical exertion,
  and asthma, 27
physical fatigue,
  with fainting, 82
pierced ears, 76
pigeon toes, 135
pigmented moles, 32, 127
pigtails,
  and baldness, 30
pimples, 22
  in shingles, 152
pinworms, 136
pityriasis rosea, 77, 137
plantar warts, 155, 183
pleurisy,
  with chest pain, 44
pleurodynia, 180
  with chest pain, 44
pneumococcal infection, 125
  in arthritis, 26
  in pneumonia, 138
pneumococci vaccine, 17
pneumonia, 17, 88, 138
  and measles, 124
  and shortness of breath, 153
  and strep throat, 161
  in cystic fibrosis, 62
  with chest pain, 44
  with toxoplasmosis, 175
pneumothorax,
  and chest pain, 44
  and shortness of breath, 153
poison ivy, 14, 15, 139
  versus sunburn, 163
poisoning, 140
  and encephalitis, 78
polio, 12, 17, 141
  viruses, 180
poliomyelitis, 141
pony tails,
  and baldness, 30
poor eyesight,
  and reading difficulties, 143
poor hearing,
  and reading difficulties, 143
port wine marks, 32
postural drainage,
  for cystic fibrosis, 62
potassium iodine,
  for asthma, 27
potassium permanganate,
  for athlete's foot, 28
prochlorperazine,
  for motion sickness, 129
prolapse of urethral lining,
  with vaginal bleeding, 178
promethazine, 14
  for motion sickness, 129
prostration,
  in blood poisoning, 34
  in chicken pox, 45
  in dysentery, 74
  in meningitis, 125
  in strep throat, 161
  with sunburn, 163
protein, 23
protruding eyeballs,

  and hyperthyroidism, 171
pseudogynecomastia, 98
pulse, rapid,
  in anemia, 23
pulse, slow,
  with concussion, 51
puncture wound, 142
  and knee pain, 120
pupils of different size,
  with concussion, 51
pus,
  in boils, 35
  in conjunctivitis, 52
  in cuts, 61
  in eye tearing, 81
pyloric stenosis, 182
pylorospasm, 182
pyrantel pamoate,
  for pinworms, 136
pyrvinium pamoate,
  for pinworms, 136

Q

Quincy, 173

R

radiation therapy,
  and scoliosis, 150
rashes,
  ammonia, 64
  contagious disease, 64
  diaper, 64
  food and drug, 64
  heat, 103
  infectious, 64
  pink, in arthritis, 26
  poison ivy, 139
  seborrhea, 64
  with chicken pox, 45
  with fifth disease, 83
  with hand, foot, and mouth disease, 99
  with head lice infestation, 101
  with infectious mononucleosis, 113
  with measles, 124
  with pityriasis rosea, 137
  with Rocky Mountain spotted fever, 145
  with rubella, 147
RBCs, see red blood cells
reaction,
  to rubella vaccine, 26
reading difficulties, 143
rectal prolapse,
  in cystic fibrosis, 62
red blood cells, 22
redness of eyes,
  with common colds, 50
  with eye tearing, 81
  with influenza, 114
  with measles, 124
  with sinusitis, 154
redness of skin,
  with boils, 35
  with burns, 42
  with diaper rash, 66
  with earring problems, 75
  with eczema, 77
  with heat rash, 103
  with hives, 108
  with ingrown toenails, 115
  with poison ivy, 139
  with rubella, 147
red patches on tongue,
  with geographic tongue, 92
red streaks

with cuts, 61
respiratory infections, 88
    with cystic fibrosis, 62
respiratory syncytial virus, 138
restlessness,
    and hyperthyroidism, 171
    rheumatic fever,
        and strep throat, 161
rheumatoid arthritis, 26
    and knee pain, 120
rhinoviruses, 180
ribs, fractured,
    with chest pain, 44
rickets, 37
rickettsialpox, 116
rifampin,
    for meningitis, 125
ringworm, 77, 144
    and baldness, 30
Rocky Mountain spotted fever, 116,
    145
Rocky Mountain spotted fever vaccine,
    17
root canal infection, 97
roseola, 12, 146
rubella, 93, 147
    in arthritis, 26
rubeola, 124
runny nose
    with fifth disease, 83
    with intestinal allergies, 117
    with measles, 124
    with roseola, 146
    with whooping cough, 184

S

Sabin vaccine, 17
salicylic acid plasters,
    for warts, 183
Salk vaccine, 17, 141
salmonella infection,
    in arthritis, 26
Sarcoptes scabei, 148
Scabies, 93, 148
scaling of earlobe,
    with earring problems, 75
scaling of skin,
    with athlete's foot, 28
    with diaper rash, 66
    with earring problems, 75
    with eczema, 77
    with pityriasis rosea, 137
    with ringworm, 144
scaphoid pads,
    for flat feet, 84
scarlatina, 161
scarlet fever, 161
scars, 22
Scheuermann's disease, 29
school phobia, 149
sclerae, 79
scoliosis, 150
scorching,
    with burns, 42
scrapes, 142, 151
scratch, 21
scratchy throat,
    with bronchitis, 40
    with common colds, 50
    with laryngitis, 121
screamer's nodes, 109
sedatives, 19
self-control, 13
sepsis,
    with jaundice, 119
septicemia, 34

Sever's disease, 155
sexual molestation,
    and vaginal bleeding, 178
shingles, 152
    with chest pain, 44
shortness of breath, 153
    in anemia, 23
    in asthma, 27
    in hypertension, 111
    in pneumothorax, 44
    with chest pain, 44
sighing,
    with tics, 172
silver sulfadiazine,
    for burns, 42
singer's nodes, 109
sinusitis, 154
    and conjunctivitis, 52
    and strep throat, 161
skull fractures,
    and dizziness, 72
sleepiness, excessive,
    and hypothyroidism, 171
sleepwalking, 132
slipped femoral epiphysis, 107
smallpox, 17
smegma, 48
sneezing,
    with common colds, 50
    with hay fever, 100
sniffing,
    with tics, 172
sodium perborate,
    for herpes simplex, 106
sore heels, 155
sore throat, 156
    and conjunctivitis, 52
    with common colds, 50
    with fifth disease, 83
    with infectious mononucleosis, 113
    with influenza, 114
    with pityriasis rosea, 137
    with pneumonia, 138
    with polio, 141
    with strep throat, 161
    with tonsillitis, 173
    with viral infection, 180
sores in the mouth,
    in hand, foot, and mouth disease, 99
    in herpes simplex, 106
spasmodic croup, 60
speaking difficulty,
    in botulism, 36
speech problems, 157
spleen enlargement, 123
splinters, 21
spotted throat,
    with strep throat, 161
sprains, 158
staphylococcal infection,
    with arthritis, 26
    with impetigo, 112
    with pneumonia, 138
    with styes, 162
staphylococcus aureus, 35, 85
steroids, 15
    for acne, 22
    for asthma, 27
    for diphtheria, 69
    for hives, 108
    for insect bites, 116
    for perleche, 134
    for Rocky Mountain spotted fever,
        145
    for shingles, 152
    for sunburn, 163

for whooping cough, 184
stiff neck,
    with concussion, 51
    with meningitis, 125
    with polio, 141
stomach ache, acute, 159
stomach ache, chronic, 160
stomach ulcers, 15
stools, dark brown or black (tarry)
        colored,
    in ulcers, 176
stools, foul,
    in cystic fibrosis, 62
stools, light-colored,
    in hepatitis 104
strabismus, external 59
strabismus, internal, 59
strawberry marks, 32
strep infections, 19
strep throat, 12, 161
streptococcal infection,
    in arthritis, 26
    in impetigo, 112
    in pneumonia, 138
stress,
    with backaches, 29
stuttering, 157
styes, 35, 162
sulfonamide,
    for diarrhea in infants, 68
    for meningitis, 125
sunburn, 163
sunken eyes,
    in dehydration, 64
sun poisoning, 15
sunscreens, choice of, 163
Sus-Phrine bronchodilator, 108
swallowed objects, 164
swallowing difficulty,
    in botulism, 36
    in epiglottitis, 60
sweating, excessive,
    and hyperthyroidism, 171
sweat test, 62
swelling
    and sore heels, 155
    in cuts, 61
    in poison ivy, 139
    of eye, 81
    of gums, 106, 123
    of hand, 70
    of salivary glands, 130
    of wrist, 70
swimmer's ear, 165
    and draining ear, 73
syncytial virus, 60
synovitis of the hip, acute, 107

T

tearing,
    in eye allergies, 79
teething, 166
temperature,
    how to take, 12
    oral, 12
    rectal, 12
tenderness,
    with backaches, 29
    with cuts, 61
    with ingrown toenails, 115
    with shingles, 152
    with sore heels, 155
    with styes, 162
    with testicles, 130
    with torsion of testicle, 167
tenderness of eyes,